The
SIX-PACK
DIET PLAN

The Secrets to Getting Lean Abs and a Rock-Hard Body Permanently

Rehan Jalali

T0273415

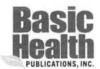

Basic Health
PUBLICATIONS, INC.

The information contained in this book is based upon the research and personal and professional experiences of the author. It is not intended as a substitute for consulting with your physician or other healthcare provider. Any attempt to diagnose and treat an illness should be done under the direction of a healthcare professional.

The publisher does not advocate the use of any particular healthcare protocol but believes the information in this book should be available to the public. The publisher and author are not responsible for any adverse effects or consequences resulting from the use of the suggestions, preparations, or procedures discussed in this book. Should the reader have any questions concerning the appropriateness of any procedures or preparation mentioned, the author and the publisher strongly suggest consulting a professional healthcare advisor.

Basic Health Publications, Inc.

Library of Congress Cataloging-in-Publication Data

Jalali, Rehan.
The six-pack diet plan : the secrets to getting lean abs and a rock-hard body permanently / Rehan Jalali.

   p. cm.
Includes bibliographical references and index.
ISBN 978-1-59120-139-7 (Pbk.)
ISBN 978-1-68162-818-9 (Hardcover)

1. Weight loss. 2. Physical fitness. I. Title.
RM222.2.J34   2004   2004018680
613.2'5—dc22

Editor: John Anderson
Copyeditor: Dana Jacoby
Typesetting/Book design: Gary A. Rosenberg
Cover design: Mike Stromberg

Contents

Acknowledgments

I would like to first and foremost thank God, most gracious, most merciful. This project would have never been completed without the support of my loving wife, Sofia, and my children, Zakir and Jayda—you are the reason why I do this. I would also like to thank my amazing and supportive parents, Kazi and Farzana Jalali, my brother, Adnan, and sisters Afia, Aisha, and Sadia, my wonderful and helpful in-laws, and my extended family in Houston and Dallas. This book is dedicated to all those people who have tried to lose fat and failed: finally, there *is* a long-term fat loss solution!

I would like to thank all the members of The Supplement Research Foundation for their support. Thanks also to all my training partners, past and present, in Texas and Southern California, including big Ray and the OC boys! I would like to thank my business partner, training partner, and friend, Millard Baker, for all his support over the last ten years. I would like to thank John Balik and *Ironman* magazine for publishing my first article a long, long time ago. Thanks to Josh Shackman, Ph.D., for providing technical assistance with the book. My problem-solving lawyer and buddy, Omar Siddiqui, and close friends Riaz Surti and David Kennedy have been a great help to me over the years. And Dr. Karlis Ullis has always provided me with good insights. Thanks to all the magazines that publish my work and perpetuate my ultimate goal of helping people achieve fitness success. This book was written for all those people who want to lose fat permanently and get lean abs without resorting to extreme fad diets and/or painful surgery.

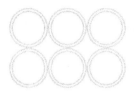

Introduction

SIX-PACK ABDOMINAL MUSCLES have long been viewed as the sign of ultimate physical fitness. The "washboard" stomach can be seen on bodybuilders, professional athletes, and advertising models. The phrase "nice six-pack" is heard echoing on beaches across the United States. But why do so many people have trouble getting lean abs and lowering their body fat? Can you get six-pack abs and maintain this level of fitness permanently?

MOST DIETS DON'T WORK

The problem is that most diets simply don't work on a long-term basis. That is why so many dieters go through the "yo-yo" effect of on again/off again weight gain and loss. Many diets are simply metabolic tricks to boost weight loss and do not address the long-term, biochemical bodily processes that are necessary for creating a lean, healthy, mirror-friendly body.

The Six-Pack Diet Plan is different. It is more than a simple diet—it's a mindset and lifestyle change. The Six-Pack Diet Plan is a long-term weight-loss solution that specifically targets problem areas like the abdominal region. This plan uses your body's natural internal components, such as hormones and other biochemicals, to help you win the battle of the bulge and create an environment in your body that is fat-loss friendly.

Most individuals who train seriously are determined to get a six-pack and eliminate that wretched abdominal fat. But many of them will fail be - cause of improper nutrition and supplementation. That stubborn abdomi-

1

nal fat is like those annoying relatives at a family barbecue—it's the last thing to go!

What's really important to know is that abdominal fat is not only detrimental to appearance but it can also be an indicator of many health risks. Research has shown that an increased amount of abdominal fat is specifically linked to hypertension, diabetes, heart disease, stroke, and high cholesterol. These risk factors associated with central body fat distribution are independent of overall obesity and can heighten its dangers even more. Scientists have also linked abdominal fat to depression, anxiety, and even social difficulties. So, getting a six-pack is not only good for looks but also beneficial for mental and physical health.

Obesity is becoming an epidemic in the United States. America may be the richest country in the world, but it is also the unhealthiest. According to recent findings by the U.S. Centers for Disease Control (CDC), 40 million adult Americans are obese and an estimated 61 percent are considered overweight. According to the U.S. Surgeon General's office, approximately 300,000 deaths a year are associated with obesity. It's no wonder that the top New Year's resolution for the past twenty years has been to lose weight.

THE FAT-LOSS PUZZLE

Everyone seems to have a "magical" solution for losing excess weight, but it's not magic that will help take the fat off. It is a combination of commitment, proper nutrition, optimal supplementation, and quality training. The Six-Pack Diet Plan offers research-based concepts to optimize each facet of the fat-loss puzzle. And like any puzzle, it takes all the pieces to make it complete. In other words, you can't just follow the nutrition portion of the plan and ignore the training aspects. It takes proper nutrition, training, supplementation, and perseverance to create a long-term fat loss solution that you can live with—a comprehensive plan such as the one detailed in this book.

After working with people from all walks of life and with all sorts of body types, I have learned some important lessons about losing fat. One thing that clearly stands out is that it definitely takes a long-term commitment to achieve permanent results. Certainly, short-term weight loss can be achieved by using many metabolic tricks, such as depleting carbohydrates and losing water weight, but this can lead to weight regain and other health problems in the long run.

The Six-Pack Diet Plan creates a healthy lifestyle that enables you to continue losing fat and maintain your desired weight. Rather than relying on metabolic tricks, it is a science-based program that addresses every aspect of long-term fat loss for achieving a healthy body. This program makes your body work for, not against, you to maximize fat burning while minimizing fat storage.

It's estimated that, after one year, over 90 percent of people who go on a diet end up a few pounds heavier than when they started. The problem is that you need to look at body fat, not body weight. People who are obsessed with overall weight tend to regain weight faster because they are using metabolic tricks to get the weight off—once your body adapts to the tricks, the results will diminish. Plus, if you lose lean muscle mass (as opposed to fat), you actually lower your metabolic rate and decrease the body's ability to lose fat. The key is to preserve lean muscle mass, lose body fat, and be happy doing it!

The Six-Pack Diet Plan uses key techniques to maximize metabolism, optimize your fat-burning hormones, boost nutrient absorption, balance blood sugar and insulin, lower fat-causing cortisol levels, and target that dreaded abdominal fat. It provides "abdominal friendly" foods and supplements that can be used to effectively reduce body fat and maintain lean body mass over the long term. It teaches you that overeating is a major fat-loss obstacle and that eating small portions of healthy foods will frequently lead to appetite control and fat loss. Even though many people see good short-term results from this program, it is meant to be a permanent fat-loss solution. Anything that is worth achieving requires effort and dedication.

A LOOK AHEAD

It may sound like a slogan, but intensity is the key to achieving extraordinary results. I mean intensity in everything—intense mindset, intense training, intense dieting, and intense supplementation. That is what it takes to achieve amazing results on this program. As the saying goes, "Only those who see the invisible can do the impossible."

But it is not impossible to get lean abs and a fat-free body in as little as eight weeks. In fact, it is more probable, if you follow the Six-Pack Diet Plan to a "T." Your body is programmed to store fat to satisfy the primitive feast/famine mechanism it uses as a survival strategy, so you must shock it into losing fat permanently. The Six-Pack Diet Plan shows you how to accomplish this for your best fat-loss results ever.

The Six-Pack Diet Plan is a revolutionary concept that combines proper eating and meal timing with key supplements and maximum, short-duration training. Leanness must be a way of life and this plan tells you how to get there fast and maintain it. The Six-Pack Diet Plan is not a theory—it is a proven plan that has worked for many people looking to lose fat permanently. In fact, I have followed this plan myself to get ready for natural bodybuilding competitions and magazine photo shoots. Being a sports nutritionist, I have to practice what I preach. As they say, you can never trust a skinny chef!

In Chapter 1: How the Body Burns Fat, we'll look at the body's mechanisms for burning off fat and how you can take advantage of these processes to increase your weight loss. You'll learn about "brown fat" and how it can actually help you lose weight; the effects of hormones on fat loss; and the importance of controlling cortisol levels in the body. In Chapter 2: The Six-Pack Eating Plan, I'll outline the foods that can help you stay lean, the importance of meal timing, and the nutrients that are helpful for burning fat. In Chapter 3: Fat-Loss Supplements, we'll look at research-based supplements, both thermogenic and non-stimulant, for helping the body burn off fat faster. Chapter 4: Hormone-Modifying Strategies explores ways to stimulate hormones in the body to lose weight safely and quickly. Chapter 5: Vitamins and Minerals for Optimal Health covers nutrients necessary to maintain healthy body function. Remember, the Six-Pack Diet Plan is not just about losing weight but living healthy as well. In Chapter 6: The Six-Pack Training Program, I'll show you the cardiovascular and weight-training program that can help turn a flabby stomach into a solid six-pack. Finally, Putting It All Together helps you incorporate all the elements of the Six-Pack Diet Plan into your life.

It's time to put your tray table up, put your seat in its upright and locked position, and get ready for some information that will radically and permanently transform your body and your life.

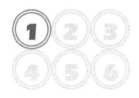

How the Body Burns Fat

O BESITY, OR GREATER FAT STORAGE, usually results from a continuous imbalance between energy intake and energy expenditure. The key to fat loss is lowering energy intake and/or increasing energy expenditure; however, it's not only about calories in and calories out.

Fat burning is a very sophisticated and detailed biochemical process. Manipulating this process is essential to your success with the Six-Pack Diet Plan. Knowing how the body burns fat and using that knowledge to your advantage is the essence of this program. Body metabolism and hormones play crucial roles in fat burning. To truly understand this complex topic, it is necessary to review how the body actually burns fat and uses it as fuel.

FAT AS FUEL

Fat contains nine calories per gram, which makes it the most energy-dense macronutrient (a gram of protein or carbohydrate contains four calories per gram). Fatty acids are stored as triglycerides (three fatty acids and one glycerol unit) in adipose (fat) tissue. Burning one gram of fat for fuel provides more energy than burning a gram of carbohydrate or protein.

Fats are oxidized (burned) to provide energy through a process called beta-oxidation (or lipolysis). When blood sugar levels are low, especially during longer periods between meals, the hormone glucagon is secreted by the pancreas and this stimulates enzyme activity to release fatty acids from triglycerides. Epinephrine (adrenaline) can stimulate the same enzymes to release energy during the stress response.

Once they are released, these fatty acids travel through the blood to other body tissues, such as muscle, where they are oxidized to provide energy through the mitochondrial beta-oxidation pathway. The mitochondria are the "furnaces" in the cells of the body. Basically, fatty acids are converted to acetyl-CoA (coenzyme-A) in this process and can then provide energy. Another destination of coenzyme-A is the production of ketone bodies by the liver, which can then provide energy to tissues like the heart and brain.

This process may increase thermogenesis, the production of heat by metabolic processes, leading to fat loss. Your metabolism is what keeps all the normal functions of your body active throughout the day and night— breathing, blood circulation, maintaining body temperature, digestion, and so on. By boosting the level of thermogenesis to accomplish all of these functions, you can burn off more fat.

Cardiovascular exercise can help mobilize fatty acid stores to be utilized as fuel. Moderate aerobic activity seems to burn more fat, although more intense cardiovascular exercise for the same duration may allow you to continue burning fat for several hours after exercise. The best time to do cardio is first thing in the morning on an empty stomach, drinking plenty of water and using a thermogenic supplement beforehand. This is when insulin levels are low and glucagon is higher, which helps prime the body for fat utilization (using fat for fuel).

The Importance of Brown Fat

There are different types of fat tissue found in humans, including white adipose tissue (white fat), which is the majority of stored fat in the body. The other, more interesting type is brown adipose tissue (BAT), which actually burns calories by using up metabolic energy to create body heat. Brown fat contains large numbers of mitochondria (the energy-producing organelle) to facilitate calorie burning. BAT is generally located deep in the body— down the spine and adjacent to the heart and kidneys.

One way to stimulate fat loss is by activating beta-adrenergic receptors (located in fat cells and activated by certain nutrients)—mainly beta-1 and beta-2. The beta-3 receptors also show great potential for fat loss. Stimulating these receptors "turns on" the fat-loss process in the corresponding cells. Beta-3 agonists (which stimulate these receptors) help target BAT, as these receptors are only found in fat tissue. Scientists have found that the beta-3 receptors are abundant in the thermogenic brown fat cells, especially within the abdominal region. It is theorized that stimulating the beta-3 receptors may help reduce abdominal fat.

BAT can also be found between the shoulder blades. So, the next time you do cardio, touch the area between your shoulder blades to feel the extra heat being produced. Many of the heat-producing effects of BAT are due to the expression of uncoupling protein-1 (UCP-1) gene. UCP-1 is exclusively found in the mitochondria of brown fat cells (white fat cells do not have mitochondria). You can think of UCP-1 as the light that ignites the fat-burning flame in fat cells. Certain nutrients (like conjugated linoleic acid) can increase UCP-1 to further enhance fat loss.

By finding ways to activate brown adipose tissue—the mitochondrial furnaces—body fat can be reduced, especially in problem areas like the abdomen.

THE THERMIC EFFECT OF FOOD

Another important factor affecting fat loss is the thermic effect of food. You might have noticed that after eating a large meal, you sometimes feel warm or even sweaty. This is due to the thermic (or heat-producing) effect of food as you digest it. Whenever your body temperature is higher, you are burning more calories. Eating frequent small meals of the right type of foods can actually be one way to boost your metabolism and burn more fat, precisely because of this thermic effect.

But keep in mind that not all foods are created equal when it comes to the thermic effect. For example, calories from fat have almost no thermic effect. Your body can store fat very easily without using much energy, hence little or no thermic effect. However, protein is very difficult to convert to fat, so it has a very large thermic effect, as high as 30 percent. What this means is that if you eat 100 calories of protein, 30 calories will be burned just as heat so that your body can digest the protein. Other research indicates that a high-protein, low-fat meal boosts post-meal thermogenesis by 100 percent compared to a high-carbohydrate, low-fat meal. That's why protein is an essential macronutrient in the Six-Pack Diet Plan, which uses the thermic effect of food to enhance metabolism and fat-burning day and night.

THE HORMONE LINK

Many people complain that they just can't lose weight, in spite of dieting, performing "lung-burning" cardio sessions, and taking handfuls of supplements. The solution may be inside you—it's all about your own hormones.

When trying to get as lean as possible and drop weight, you must consider ways to maximize your body's natural hormones to more effectively influence fat burning. These powerful substances can mean the difference between a lean, fit body and a fat, unhealthy one.

Hormones are biologically active substances that regulate many key processes throughout the body. "Nothing can influence our body's shape more than our own hormones . . . Hormones regulate weight, metabolism, how much muscle we have, food intake, and many other factors," says Karlis Ullis, M.D., noted hormone expert and author of *The Hormone Revolution Weight Loss Plan.* There are some key hormones with regard to fat loss and muscle gain: the major players include growth hormone (GH), the sex hormones testosterone and estrogen, the thyroid hormones, insulin, and cortisol. "Without taking into account our hormones and how we exercise, we predictably will regain all the weight we lost on some 'crash diet' plan," states Dr. Ullis.

By learning to optimize the effects of these key hormones, you can maximize your fitness routine and lose weight. Hormones can be powerful allies in your battle to achieve a great physique. The Six-Pack Diet Plan addresses each hormone and helps these hormones to work synergistically in your fat-loss efforts.

Growth Hormone

Human growth hormone (GH) is the most abundant hormone produced by the pituitary gland. It is mainly released in pulses during sleep and GH secretion usually decreases with age. Most of growth hormone's powerful effects are due to its conversion in the liver to IGF-1 (insulin-like growth factor type 1). IGF-1 is actually what is measured in a blood test to determine GH levels in the body.

Growth hormone has been shown to increase lean body mass, reduce body fat, increase energy, stimulate immune function, and even enhance sexual function. GH enhances protein metabolism and other processes and this is mediated by IGF-1. IGF-1 boosts muscle and bone mass and it has important effects on carbohydrate, protein, and bone metabolism. It stimulates cell replication, cell differentiation, and the synthesis of cellular products. In diabetics, IGF-1 increases insulin sensitivity and improves glucose utilization, which can reduce fat storage. Obesity diminishes the release of GH, while fasting actually helps increase it.

Because GH is released primarily during sleep, it is important to get sufficient amounts of sleep every night. Exercise, both cardiovascular and weight training, is a potent stimulus for GH release. Diet can also affect GH levels. For example, a study published in the *Journal of Nutrition* in 2002 showed that men consuming soy protein isolate (40 grams daily) had increased levels of IGF-1. The Six-Pack Diet Plan helps you use growth hormone to stimulate fat loss and support lean body mass.

Testosterone and Estrogen

Testosterone is a sex (steroid) hormone produced by the testes and adrenal glands that promotes the development of male sex characteristics and regulates male reproductive function. It is called the most powerful muscle-building hormone because it does just that—builds muscle and strength fast. Testosterone increases muscle protein synthesis and net muscle protein balance, resulting in increased muscle mass. "Testosterone is one of the most effective hormones for burning fat in both men and women," states Dr. Ullis.

Signs of low testosterone levels include low energy, muscle weakness, depression, and sexual dysfunction. However, too much testosterone in males can also cause problems—it may convert into DHT (dihydrotestosterone), which can have adverse effects on the prostate gland and cause hair loss. It can also convert into estrogen, leading to water retention and increased fat storage. A diet rich in essential fatty acids and certain types of weight training exercises can help boost testosterone levels.

It is important to measure both "free testosterone" levels (the active form) and estrogen levels in order to make sure there is not too much estrogen being produced. Estrogen can literally halt your muscle-building efforts. Estrogen is one of the body's most powerful fat-storage hormones and higher estrogen levels in men can cause abdominal fat storage, bloating, and fatigue. Make sure you don't have any mineral deficiencies, such as calcium or zinc, as this may be linked to high estrogen. Drinking green tea and eating flaxseed may help lower estrogen levels as well.

Thyroid Hormones

When people are trying to lose weight, they often experience a decrease in basal metabolic rate (BMR), which represents the number of calories that are burned at rest. This is especially true after long periods of low-calorie dieting, the use of stimulants (including caffeine), and excessive amounts of physical activity. The body seems to reduce metabolism as a defense mechanism. That is why some people following these types of weight-loss regimes claim they cannot lose that last bit of fat.

The decrease in BMR is directly related to the level of thyroid hormones. Thyroid hormone activity is defined by the levels of two hormones released by the thyroid gland, thyroxine (T4) and triiodothyronine (T3). T4 is a low-activity hormone and T3 is a highly active thyroid hormone. T4 converts into T3 in the liver. Thyroid hormones are important for growth and development, as well as for maintaining metabolism and normal body weight. Thyroid hormones also exert effects on thermogenesis and temperature regulation and can enhance lipolysis (fat burning) in adipose tissue.

To determine if your thyroid hormones are imbalanced, it is important to test T3 levels, since this is the most active hormone. The diet, weight training, and nutritional therapy components of the Six-Pack Diet Plan can influence the metabolism and activity of thyroid hormones.

Insulin

Insulin is a hormone produced in the beta cells of the pancreas. It is released due to a rise in blood sugar (glucose) levels in the body, which is induced mainly by eating carbohydrates. This hormone is primarily responsible for the direction of energy metabolism after eating; it can help transport key nutrients like glucose and amino acids into muscle cells, but it can also cause fat storage to occur.

Many people talk about controlling blood sugar, and hence insulin, levels to prevent fat storage, reduce cravings, and sustain energy levels. Other diets may have you eliminate carbohydrates altogether to minimize and control insulin levels. But can insulin really help you build more muscle mass or does it just cause more fat storage and halt your fat-loss goals? Insulin has been discussed heavily in the health and dieting communities and is a vital hormone in the Six-Pack Diet Plan. It's time to set the record straight and find out more about this intriguing hormone. (And, yes, you *can* positively manipulate it.)

Insulin helps regulate blood sugar levels and keeps them in the normal range. Normal fasting blood glucose levels should be 70–110 mg/dl (milligrams per deciliter). Individuals with type I diabetes cannot produce insulin, so insulin shots are necessary. In type II diabetes, they cannot use their insulin properly and may have insulin insensitivity. Insulin binds to specific receptors in cell membranes and helps drive glucose into the cells. Normally the cell membranes are impermeable to glucose, but when a cell receptor is activated, the membrane allows for a rapid entry of glucose into the cells. Insulin also activates glycogen synthase, an enzyme that helps glycogen (the stored form of glucose) to be stored in muscle tissue and the liver. Liver glycogen is mainly used to help keep blood sugar levels stable.

Insulin allows cell membranes to become more permeable to certain amino acids, creatine, and some minerals. Insulin causes glucose transporter proteins (GLUT) to increase their activity, allowing for increased glucose uptake by muscle cells during exercise. Two of these proteins are found in skeletal muscle: GLUT 1, which is present in low levels, and GLUT 4, which is responsible for the increase in glucose transport in response to insulin and muscle contractions.

It is believed that both insulin and exercise stimulate an increase of GLUT 4 transporters in the plasma membrane of skeletal muscle. Both exercise (muscle contraction, to be specific) and insulin stimulate an increase in glucose uptake by muscle; however, there is ample evidence suggesting that exercise during muscle recovery impedes glycogen synthesis. This is why I recommend that you refrain from any cardiovascular work right after resistance training—it may inhibit glycogen resynthesis and not allow your body to recover from your weight-training session properly.

Although insulin helps dispose of blood glucose by storing it as glycogen, it can also convert the excess sugar into fat. Insulin is truly a double-edged sword because of this effect. What many people don't know is that insulin supports amino acid uptake into muscle tissue as well, helping in the growth and recovery process after exercise. Enhancing glycogen levels in the muscle cells creates a more favorable environment for growth. It also causes cellular swelling (for every gram of glycogen stored in the muscle cell, there are 3 grams of water stored as well), which can have a hydrating effect on the muscle and create more stored energy to be used later.

Insulin's opposing hormone is glucagon, which is activated when blood sugar levels are too low. This hormone can break down muscle tissue and reduce glycogen stores, so it is important to control it as well.

What and when you eat can have a profound effect on your insulin levels—the Six-Pack Diet Plan can help you maximize the benefits of insulin. A wide array of supplements is available to naturally balance blood sugar and insulin levels. Plus, some athletes report a better muscular "pump" when using insulin-boosting supplements.

The Cortisol Factor

Most people have heard of cortisol and many know that it's bad news. Unfortunately, they don't know the extent of damage this hormone can cause, especially when they are trying to get lean abs. This muscle-wasting hormone literally eats away at fat-loss potential.

Cortisol is the primary glucocorticoid, a natural hormone produced by the adrenal glands (located atop the kidneys). Although cortisol's precise actions are not completely understood, we know that it is essential for life. It is necessary to maintain important processes (heart rate, blood pressure, adrenaline release) in times of stress. Most of its effects are not directly responsible for the initiation of metabolic or circulatory processes, but it is necessary for their full response.

Normal kidney function also requires cortisol. When there is an absence or deficiency of cortisol, water cannot be excreted rapidly, which can consequently lead to water retention. (This may also occur with too much cortisol.) Controlling cortisol levels, and thus lowering excess body water and abdominal fat, is one of the ways the Six-Pack Diet Plan can make you look leaner. (We will get to cortisol and its effects on abdominal fat in just a little while.)

What Causes Excess Cortisol?

Any type of stress that occurs to the body signals the nervous system to relay this to the hypothalamus. The hypothalamus then responds by initiating the "stress hormone cascade," starting with corticotrophin-releasing hormone (CRH), followed by adrenocorticotropic hormone (ACTH) release, and finally glucocorticoid (cortisol) production. Stress to the human body can include trauma, anxiety, infections, surgery, and even resistance training and aerobics.

Recent research has shown that elevated cortisol levels increased protein breakdown by 5 to 20 percent. Even mild elevations in cortisol can increase blood glucose concentration and protein catabolism (muscle breakdown) within a few hours in healthy individuals. Cortisol can also increase body fat, especially when the level of cortisol rises dramatically in the body.

Overtraining by athletes may cause higher cortisol levels, potentially leading to hypertension, because cortisol causes sodium retention and potassium excretion. Excess cortisol causes insulin resistance by decreasing the rate at which insulin activates the glucose uptake system. Cortisol levels rise as you increase the amount of time devoted to intense exercise. In overtrained individuals, cortisol levels increase while testosterone levels decrease. That is why one measure of overtraining is the testosterone:cortisol ratio.

The Unhealthy Effects of Cortisol

Cortisol reduces the utilization of amino acids for protein formation in muscle cells. A cortisol excess can lead to a progressive loss of protein, muscle weakness and atrophy, and loss of bone mass through increased calcium excretion and decreased calcium absorption. The major catabolic (muscle breakdown) effects of cortisol involve facilitating the conversion of protein in muscles and connective tissue into glucose and glycogen. This involves both the increased degradation of protein already formed and the decreased synthesis of new protein. Cortisol can also decrease the utilization of glucose through directly inhibiting glucose transport into the cells. A cortisol excess can lead to a decrease in insulin sensitivity and adversely affect tendon health by weakening them.

Excess cortisol causes a redistribution of body fat to occur through an unknown mechanism. Basically, the extremities lose fat and muscle while the trunk and face become fatter. Several studies have verified that high cortisol levels are directly linked with increased abdominal fat and can even cause binge eating (especially sweets). One study published in *Obesity Research Journal* clearly showed that men with higher levels of cortisol had greater abdominal fat deposits. Another study in *Psychoneuroendocrinology* suggested that women with high stress levels (which increases cortisol) ate more calories and consumed a greater amount of sweet foods. This study linked high cortisol levels to binge eating in women. The scientists conducting the study concluded that this pattern could adversely impact body weight and health over the long run. Researchers from the University of California, San Francisco, in another study published in *Psychosomatic Medicine,* stated that "central fat distribution is related to greater psychological vulnerability to stress and cortisol reactivity." Abdominal fat is especially sensitive to the fat-accumulating effects of cortisol, because it has four times more receptors for cortisol than fat found elsewhere in the body. So, if you want to get lean, especially in the abdominal area, you have to control cortisol levels.

Cortisol inhibits growth hormone levels by stimulating the release of somatostatin, a growth hormone antagonist (inhibitor). It may also reduce IGF-1 expression. IGF-1 is one of the most anabolic (muscle-building) agents in the body and is the substance responsible for most of the positive effects of growth hormone.

Cortisol has other hormone-modifying effects. It can directly inhibit gonadotropin, which is produced by the pituitary, and TSH (thyroid-stimulating hormone). By doing so, cortisol makes the target tissues of sex steroids and growth factors resistant to these substances. It may also suppress an enzyme that converts the relatively inactive thyroid hormone T4 into the active form T3 (triiodothyronine), which can decrease the metabolic rate and make it harder to lose body fat.

Cortisol also seems to play a role in various diseases. It is found in higher levels in diseases ranging from AIDS and multiple sclerosis to Alzheimer's disease. Prolonged high levels of cortisol can throw the immune system into chaos and ravage the human body. A growing number of researchers believe that many of the worst, and least understood, diseases will soon be identified as caused by high cortisol, and subsequently treated with cortisol-reducing drugs or supplements.

The Six-Pack Diet Plan can help you control cortisol levels so that you can reduce body fat and build lean, strong muscles.

HOW THE SIX-PACK DIET PLAN HELPS BURN FAT

As you can see, fat burning is very complex, but the Six-Pack Diet Plan can help you use these myriad processes to your advantage. In the following chapters, we'll explore diet, nutritional supplements, and training methods that can help you lose weight and get a defined physique. What you eat and the timing of meals can modify insulin and help speed up your metabolism. A number of supplements, training tips, and other strategies can increase fat burning and modify hormone levels. The Six-Pack Diet Plan works with your body's natural processes to maximize weight loss and muscle building.

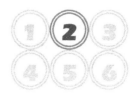

The Six-Pack Eating Plan

T
O BUILD YOUR BEST BODY EVER, it takes a combination of proper nutrition, training, and supplementation, with nutrition being the most important of the three components. The problem is figuring out how to eat properly in order to get a lean body and maintain it permanently.

To start the discussion about eating for leanness, it is important to review the basic components of food and their effects on the body. Whole foods (that is, foods in their natural nutrient-rich form) provide protein, carbohydrates (including sugar and fiber), and fat (saturated and unsaturated essential fatty acids). Each of these foods is important for maintaining a healthy, fit body.

It's not just what you eat that's important, but also when you eat. The timing of certain meals can help you burn off more fat and build more muscle. Also, by eating small meals throughout the day instead of three big meals, you can more evenly balance your blood sugar and insulin, improve nutrient absorption, and take advantage of the thermic effect of food.

Convenience is always a big part of sticking with a diet program. This chapter will also cover recommendations for using meal-replacement powders and protein bars with the Six-Pack Diet Plan.

PROTEIN

Protein, which provides four calories of energy per gram, is the building block of muscle and amino acids are the building blocks of protein. There are essential amino acids, ones you must get from the diet because your body cannot produce them (tryptophan, lysine, methionine, phenylalanine, threonine, valine, leucine, and isoleucine), and non-essential amino acids (such as tyrosine, glycine, cysteine, proline, serine, and aspartic acid).

Protein helps support lean muscle tissue, aids in the production of hormones and enzymes, and supports immune function. Exercising individuals have higher daily protein requirements than sedentary individuals as exercise increases the body's need for protein. Since protein is necessary to build muscle, it can actually help speed up metabolism, because it takes energy (calories) to maintain lean muscle mass at rest. This may allow you to lose more fat.

Recommended Proteins

- **Whey protein**—This highly absorbable protein provides the highest concentration of the BCAAs (branched chain amino acids) leucine, isoleucine, and valine, which play a key role in the muscle-building process and also support immune function. Hydrolyzed whey protein has some of the benefits of whey while providing highly absorbable peptides that can have anabolic (muscle-building) effects.

- **Casein**—A milk protein that seems to have a timed-release effect and a high glutamine content, which can enhance exercise recovery and boost immune function. Clinically proven to increase lean muscle mass and strength, casein is a good nighttime protein.

- **Milk protein isolate**—This contains both whey and casein and is a good source for these two proteins.

- **Soy protein isolate**—This vegetarian protein source has been shown to enhance thyroid hormone output, which can increase metabolic rate to support fat loss. The isoflavones in soy have numerous health benefits, including lowering cholesterol and triglyceride levels. It contains an excellent ratio of glutamine, arginine, and BCAAs. Soybeans, tofu, soymilk, and other forms of soy contain some soy protein concentrate, which is not the same thing as soy protein isolate. Soy foods can actually be estrogenic in men and cause water retention and bloating.

- **Egg albumin**—This traditional protein source boasts a great amino acid profile. Cooked egg whites are a good source of egg albumin.

- **Chicken breast**—A relatively low-fat, high-quality protein source, chicken contains high doses of BCAAs and has a good potassium-to-sodium ratio (which can positively influence water balance).

- **Top sirloin steak**—A lean protein source with an excellent potassium-to-sodium ratio, it provides heme iron and good amounts of the amino acids alanine and lysine, which can support energy and lean body mass.

- **Tuna**—This is another lean protein source that provides an excellent amount of BCAAs. Canned versions make it easy to use and help with portion control.

- **Orange roughy fish**—A very lean protein source with an outstanding potassium-to-sodium ratio, orange roughy is a good source of the amino acids leucine and lysine.

Other quality food sources of protein include salmon, mahi mahi, sword-fish, skim milk (occasionally), and black beans (for vegetarians).

Carbohydrates

Carbohydrates are the major source of energy for humans, providing four calories per gram. There are several types of carbohydrates, including simple sugars, complex carbohydrates, and dietary fiber. Carbohydrates support energy levels in the body and also can have a protein-sparing effect.

The glycemic index is a rating of carbohydrates and their effect on blood sugar levels. The higher the glycemic index of a certain carbohydrate, the greater the blood sugar response after eating it. High blood sugar responses to foods can cause fat storage to occur and "yo-yo" energy levels. Consuming dietary fiber or protein with a carbohydrate can lower the glycemic rating.

Carbohydrates are stored in the liver and muscle tissue as glycogen. Eating lower glycemic index carbohydrates can allow for a steady release of energy and help keep blood sugar levels stable. Lower glycemic carbs like sweet potatoes and multi-grain oatmeal are six-pack friendly carbs.

Also, the more processed the food—most convenience foods—the higher its glycemic index (thereby speeding its entrance into the bloodstream). For example, instant rice has a higher glycemic rating than slow-cooked rice. Fruit is very interesting in that it provides a form of carbo-hydrate called fructose. This is a low-glycemic carbohydrate but since it is metabolized primarily in the liver, it can slow down metabolism and may cause fat storage to occur if eaten in excess.

But as good as the glycemic index is for rating the effects of carbohydrates on blood sugar, it is deficient because it doesn't address the issue of mixed meals. In other words, when you eat a meal containing protein along with carbohydrates (such as a tuna sandwich), the glycemic (and blood sugar) response will be much lower. The same holds true for mixing carbohydrates with fat or dietary fiber. On the Six-Pack Diet Plan, there are times when simple carbs are allowed, even encouraged, but in general it is best to eat mixed meals to lower the glycemic response.

• • • SIX-PACK DIET APPROVED CARBOHYDRATES • • •		
Complex	**Fibrous**	**Simple**
Oatmeal	Asparagus	Dates
Multi-grain oatmeal	Broccoli	Raisins
Yam	Cabbage	Grapefruit
Sweet potato	Cauliflower	Banana
White rice	Corn	Apple juice
Brown rice	Green beans	Blueberries
Black beans	Tomato	Honey, raw
White potato	Lettuce	Corn chips, unsalted

Fiber

During the last twenty years, research has proven that dietary fiber is important for gastrointestinal function and the prevention of disease. Dietary fiber is defined as "plant polysaccharides and lignin, which are resistant to hydrolysis by the digestive enzymes in man." In other words, fiber remains intact through the gastrointestinal tract, thus having a cleansing function. Insoluble fibers include lignin, cellulose, and some hemicellulose. Soluble fibers include pectin, gum, mucilages, and some hemi-cellulose. Healthy effects of fiber include increased fecal bulk, the reduction of colon cancer, delayed gastric emptying, reduced glucose absorption (lowers glycemic index of foods), and detoxification. Many dieters and exercising individuals are lacking in daily fiber intake. With the Six-Pack Diet Plan, you will be consuming plenty of fiber, especially at night, to keep your metabolism going.

Recommended Sources of Fiber

Quality fiber sources include oatmeal and multi-grain oatmeal, flaxseeds, beans (kidney, black, red, navy, pinto, and garbanzo), figs, almonds, peanuts, broccoli, peas, dates, prunes, and raisins.

Larch arabinogalactan (AG) is a polysaccharide powder derived from the wood of the larch tree. It is a soluble fiber that has been clinically shown to boost immune function and is particularly effective at increasing beneficial intestinal microflora, such as bifidobacteria and lactobacillus, which can help improve digestive function. This compound is well tolerated and provides an excellent source of fiber. Since AG is virtually tasteless and mixes easily, it can be added to a meal-replacement shake to boost fiber content. Taking 5–15 grams (g) daily can be very effective. AG is made by a company called Larex.

Fats

After being indoctrinated about the evils of dietary fat by nutritionists and so-called diet gurus for the last thirty years, we are now learning about the benefits of fats, especially for exercising individuals and athletes. Supplying nine calories per gram, fats provide energy to the body and essential fats, which can help support hormone levels, neurological function, and cell membrane stability.

There are saturated and unsaturated fats. Saturated fats are the ones you generally want to avoid because of their detrimental effects in the body, such as cardiovascular problems (heart disease and increased cholesterol). Saturated fats include trans fats (partially hydrogenated and hydrogenated oils), animal fats, palm oil, and coconut oil.

Unsaturated fats include the essential fatty acids (EFAs)—omega-3s (alpha-linolenic) and omega-6s (linoleic). These EFAs cannot be made by the body and must be taken in through foods or supplementation. The positive benefits of EFAs include decreasing catabolism (muscle breakdown); increasing growth hormone secretion; improving the action of insulin; enhancing oxygen utilization and energy transformation required for optimal performance; decreasing total cholesterol and increasing HDL (the so-called good cholesterol); boosting testosterone production; supporting liver function and immune function; and improving nitrogen retention. These are all great effects for individuals on a diet and fitness program.

EFAs and Prostaglandins

There's a class of hormone-like substances called prostaglandins in the body that are derived from essential fatty acids. Certain prostaglandins are beneficial for health and disease prevention, while others are part of the body's reaction to stress or injury.

There are three classes (or series) of prostaglandins. Series 1 prostaglandins, particularly PGE1, have many beneficial effects for athletes: they appear to have anabolic effects, promote thermogenesis, increase sodium and water clearance by the kidneys, and prevent blood clots. Series 2 prostaglandins have the opposite effects. They seem to trigger the release of energy substrates by breaking down structural protein, causing salt and water retention, and promoting the clotting of blood. They are useful in a fight-or-flight stress situation, when your body reacts to ensure your short-term survival by elevating your blood pressure and making energy more available.

Both series 1 and series 2 prostaglandins are derived from the same precursor, linoleic acid (an omega-6 fatty acid), while the last class, series 3 prostaglandins, are derived from linolenic acid (an omega-3 fatty acid). The series 3 prostaglandins are important not for their actions but rather for their ability to decrease the rate at which series 2 prostaglandins are formed.

So, series 1 prostaglandins promote performance, series 2 prostaglandins disrupt performance, and series 3 prostaglandins block the formation of series 2 prostaglandins. The idea is to consume EFAs that help produce series 1 and series 3 prostaglandins.

Because prostaglandins are not true hormones, they're only active in or near the cell where they're generated. True hormones move throughout the body to reach distant target organs or tissues. The downside to the local-action-only feature is that prostaglandins aren't orally bioavailable—unless you take them in huge amounts—and can only be administered intravenously. The upside is that you can take the precursors—the essential fatty acids—and still give your body the building blocks necessary to form the good prostaglandins naturally.

Recommended Essential Fat Sources

- All-natural peanut butter (PowerButter is a good brand that also provides extra protein)
- Sunflower seeds (unsalted)
- Walnuts
- Almonds
- Olive oil

- Sunflower oil

- Flaxseed oil

- Peanuts

- Fish oils—EPA and DHA (found in fish such as salmon, tuna, and orange roughy)

Water

Hydration is an important aspect of the Six-Pack Diet Plan. Water is a very underrated but essential nutrient in a fitness program. It has many functions in the body, including getting rid of toxins, transporting nutrients, promoting cellular hydration or cell volumization (which can lead to an anabolic environment inside muscle cells), and supporting healthy skin function. According to some research, dehydrating a muscle by as little as 3 percent can lead to a 12 percent decrease in strength. Plus, your muscle cells are about 70 percent water. It is important to drink one gallon of pure water daily on the Six-Pack Diet Plan. You should have clear urine as a sign that you are consuming an adequate amount of water daily.

CALORIES AND MACRONUTRIENT RATIOS

Since the Six-Pack Diet Plan addresses long-term fat loss and how to maintain lean abs permanently, counting calories is not essential. What is more important is the ratio of protein, carbohydrates, and fats eaten daily.

It is critical to eat fewer calories than you are expending. Both men and women should consume ten calories per pound of body weight each day. For example, if you are a 200-pound male, you will need to consume around 2,000 calories, separated into many small meals, daily. The Six-Pack Diet consists of 45 percent protein, 40 percent carbohydrates, and 15 percent essential fats. Here's how it breaks down:

Total Calories:

200 (pounds) $\times$ 10 (calories) = 2,000 calories consumed daily

Protein:

45 percent protein = 2,000 $\times$ 0.45 = 900 total calories from protein daily

900 calories of protein/4 calories per gram of protein = 225 grams (g) protein daily

Six-Pack Diet Restaurant Eating Guide

○ After ordering a meal, ask for a to-go box and box half your meal before you begin eating.

○ Always eat mixed meals containing a good source of protein—don't eat carbs alone.

○ At restaurants that have chefs, you can always make substitutions—ask for the steamed vegetables instead of the Caesar salad or try sweet potatoes instead of mashed potatoes. Chefs can also make alterations to your entrees. For example, ask for no oil and less salt and choose grilled versus fried foods. Ask the waiter to prepare your meal "dry," without the fatty, high-sodium extras.

○ Drink plenty of water with every meal. Avoid sodas and so-called healthier sugar-filled alternatives like juices.

○ Eat a salad before your meal and use fat-free dressing or lemon juice (and only use a small amount of that).

○ If you have to eat fast food, order a salad and grilled chicken sandwich. Then discard the bun and put the grilled chicken on the salad.

○ Watch out for calorie- and fat-filled sauces and dressings. To add flavor to your food, use cayenne pepper, lemon, garlic, ginger, or other herbs instead.

○ If you must have salty tasting food, carry a salt substitute with you, such as potassium chloride, to add to your restaurant meals.

Carbohydrates:

40 percent carbohydrates = 2,000 × 0.40 = 800 total calories from carbohydrates

800 calories of carbohydrates/4 calories per gram of carbohydrates = 200 g carbs daily

TIP: Remember to consume a good portion of these carbs first thing in the morning and after a hard workout.

Fat:

15 percent fat = 2,000 × .15 = 300 total calories from fat daily

300 calories of fat ÷ 9 calories per gram of fat = 33 g fat daily

THE IMPORTANCE OF MEAL TIMING

Meals should be eaten every 1.5 to 2 hours. Eat bigger meals in the morning and decrease calories per meal as the day progresses, so the smallest meal is your last meal. For sample meal plans, see Appendix A.

There are three very important times for food intake on the Six-Pack Diet Plan: breakfast ("morning delight"), post-workout ("the power hour"), and pre-bedtime ("night food"). Eating the right foods during these special times is essential to losing fat and maintaining lean body mass.

Breakfast: Morning Delight

Breakfast is very important because it sets a metabolic trend for your body for the coming day. You have just had an overnight fast (while sleeping) and your body is ready for nutrients. Your metabolic rate is also higher in the morning, so more calories can and should be consumed during this time.

For men, another important thing to remember is that testosterone levels are higher in the morning. Testosterone is *the* muscle-building hormone. Providing enough protein during the first meal of the day can allow maximization of testosterone output to support the building of lean muscle mass. Both men and women can benefit from protein in the morning.

Sample breakfast meals might be 8–10 egg whites with one cup of cooked oatmeal and one medium banana. A meal-replacement powder along with one cup of oatmeal and a banana also works for breakfast. Remember, this is the biggest meal of the day.

Post-Workout: The Power Hour

Post-workout is by far the most important time of the day for anyone who is trying to build a better body. What you do in the one to four hours following a workout can determine what kind of gains you will make in building your physique and if you will get leaner, stronger, and more muscular.

The greatest nutrient uptake occurs after a hard weight-training workout. It makes sense; you've depleted nutrients and now the body is ready to replenish them. Some experts even recommend consuming 50 percent of your total daily calories within the two to four hours after a hard workout.

There are several factors and reasons why nutrient absorption is heightened significantly post-workout. First, insulin sensitivity is greatest after a workout. It is critical to maximize insulin levels to drive nutrients into muscle cells. Insulin helps transport nutrients like glucose, amino acids, and creatine into muscle cells. Insulin can also cause fat storage with excess calories. When insulin sensitivity is increased most of the glucose and amino acids transported by insulin go right to the muscle cells so that fat storage is minimized. Glucose, taken up rapidly by the muscle cells following exercise, causes glycogen production and greater carbohydrate storage in muscle tissue.

The key post-workout goal is to boost muscle anabolism (increase protein synthesis, while decreasing or minimizing muscle breakdown). Lowering cortisol, replenishing glycogen stores, providing amino acids and carbohydrates in the optimum ratio (3:1 or 4:1) for maximum glycogen replenishment, and increasing cell volume to create a greater anabolic environment are all very important for building muscle mass.

The post-workout "power hour" allows you to take in more carbs at the peak time. Research has clearly demonstrated that muscle glycogen synthesis is twice as rapid if carbohydrates are consumed immediately after exercise as opposed to waiting a few hours. This is actually an approved time to consume additional simple carbohydrates (such as raisins, dates, and other simple sugars) that you may be craving. Combining protein with carbohydrates right after a workout can further enhance glycogen synthesis. In fact, a protein and carbohydrate drink can maximize insulin levels for several hours following weight training.

The addition of the amino acid L-arginine to a carbohydrate supplement post-exercise increases the availability of glucose for muscle glycogen storage. One of the reasons glycogen synthesis is enhanced after a workout is because the enzyme responsible for glycogen production (glycogen synthase) is more active and glucose transporters in muscle cells (like GLUT 4) are also active. The protein synthesis machinery of muscle cells is activated in a greater way. That is why consuming protein post-workout can help enhance protein synthesis, muscle repair, and amino acid availability.

Drinking water at this time is also important to help enhance cell volumization and transport nutrients in the body. Taking a post-workout drink is essential to proper workout recovery and muscle building.

Post-Workout: Supplement Strategy

- **Protein/Carb Drink**—This drink should be taken immediately after exercise and consist of a 3:1 carbohydrate-to-protein ratio (about 75 g carbs and 25 g protein). The protein should be from high-quality whey protein isolate, while the carbohydrates should consist of simple sugars with a high glycemic index, such as dextrose, glucose, and maltodextrin. Whey protein isolate contains a high dose of BCAAs and essential amino acids and is readily absorbed by the body. Remember, timing is everything; in the post-workout period it is important to get amino acids into muscle tissues. Consume 20–40 grams of whey protein isolate during this time.

Many research studies validate the use of a post-workout recovery drink. One study published in the *Journal of Physiology* states that "early intake of an oral protein supplement after resistance exercise is important for the development of hypertrophy in skeletal muscle." In other words, it helps build bigger muscles.

Carbohydrate supplementation right after a workout and again one hour later can decrease muscle breakdown and create a more positive body protein balance. New research indicates that consuming a protein/carbohydrate drink immediately after a workout can even increase RMR (resting metabolic rate), boosting metabolism and helping with fat loss. So, make sure you have a post-workout drink ready every time you train. Consume 16 ounces of this drink right after a workout and then another one hour after training, with additional protein and carbohydrates (a meal-replacement powder is a great choice).

- **Glutamine**—Glutamine is the most abundant amino acid in muscle tissue. Supplemental glutamine can help promote cell volumization (the drawing of water inside muscle cells, thus creating a more anabolic environment for growth). It can also increase protein synthesis, and decrease proteolysis (muscle breakdown), while partially determining the rate of protein turnover in muscles. Glutamine peptide is better absorbed than free-form glutamine (the speed of nutrient uptake is essential after training). Wheat protein hydrolysate, a common source for glutamine peptide, has been shown to increase glycogen synthesis after exercise when compared to a placebo and a free-form glutamine drink.

  Research from the Swedish University of Agricultural Sciences showed that glutamine concentration is 10 percent higher in type II (fast-twitch) muscle fibers versus type I (slow-twitch) fibers. Fast-twitch muscle fibers have a large disposition for growth and are positively affected by weight training. The same researchers showed a 45 percent decrease in glutamine in both fiber types after exercise, hence the need for supplementation. A typical dose is 5–10 g of glutamine or glutamine peptide consumed right after a workout and another 5 g one-and-a-half hours after training.

- **Branched chain amino acids (BCAAs)**—These special amino acids have been shown to act directly to potentiate protein synthesis, lower muscle breakdown, spare protein, and enhance overall recovery. A whey protein isolate supplement has plenty of BCAAs. Supplementation with higher doses of BCAAs may be useful. Five to 10 grams of BCAAs is a good start, but you can take upward of 50 grams daily. Any excess will generally be excreted.

- **Arginine**—This amino acid helps regulate protein synthesis, nitric oxide production, and immune function, and can even release growth hormone at high doses. Take 2–4 grams within thirty minutes after a workout.

- *Rhodiola rosea*—This adaptogenic herb has been shown to reduce stress and enhance the recovery process secondary to exercise. It may even modify cortisol levels. Taking 100–200 milligrams (mg) after a workout may be beneficial.

- **Chromium polynicotinate**—Chromium can aid in weight loss and also enhance insulin sensitivity by supporting glucose tolerance factor (a compound on cells that maximize insulin usage). Taking 400 micrograms (mcg) after a workout can further enhance nutrient uptake into muscle tissue and allow insulin to work more effectively.

- **Alpha lipoic acid**—This compound is an antioxidant and it supports nutrient transport by mimicking insulin. Taking 100 mg after a workout can be helpful.

- **Fenugreek seed**—There is a very interesting amino acid that is extracted from fenugreek seeds called 4-hydroxyisoleucine. This ingredient may enhance insulin secretion (direct beta-cell stimulation, which helps release insulin from the source) and help control blood sugar levels. Again, this can allow for greater transport of key nutrients, like creatine, amino acids, and glucose, into muscle tissue. A typical dose is around 300 mg twice daily with meals, one dose right after a workout.

- **Vitamins C and E**—These antioxidants can help scavenge free radicals after a workout. Free radicals delay the recovery process and damage muscle cells. Taking 500 mg of vitamin C and 400 International Units (IU) of vitamin E after a workout can speed recovery and enhance overall health.

This may seem like a lot of supplements, but keep in mind that some nutritional products contain many of these ingredients in an all-in-one formula (such as Myoplex Sport, Endurox R4, and Countdown). Also, every ingredient listed is not essential to recovery, so feel free to choose which ones you prefer for post-workout recuperation.

Pre-Bedtime: Night Food

Pre-bedtime nutrition should be considered an essential part of a weight-training and physique-changing program. The Six-Pack Diet Plan recommends key nutrients to take before bedtime to optimize muscle building and fat burning, and to lower muscle breakdown during sleep.

Before we dive right into the nutrition and supplementation tips, let's review how pre-bedtime nutrition can support your goals of increasing lean muscle mass and reducing body fat. First, you need to maximize (and minimize) key hormones, specifically increase growth hormone (GH) and testosterone levels, while lowering insulin and cortisol levels. Next, the body needs plenty of amino acids available for protein synthesis caused by GH and testosterone release during sleep. Hydration before bedtime is necessary so all the nutrients are used effectively and muscle cells can function optimally. Finally, you need an array of vitamins, minerals, and antioxidants to neutralize free radicals (which can interfere with recovery and repair during sleep) and provide key enzyme co-factors to support proper protein synthesis and muscle anabolism.

It is vital to lower insulin levels before sleep to maximize GH release and lower fat storage. Do not consume any carbohydrates (which can cause a release of insulin) within three hours of bedtime. For example, the last meal of the day should be mainly protein and fiber (such as a chicken breast salad) and the last "food" before bed should be a protein drink. (One good supplement is Night Pro HMP from ASR.) Even pure whey protein isolate can cause an insulin response, so it may be beneficial to eat a mixed protein meal (along with fiber) before bedtime.

The importance of taking protein before bedtime cannot be overstated. Since protein synthesis and breakdown occurs during sleep, it is vital to provide the body with a plethora of amino acids by taking a protein drink before sleep. Research shows that consuming amino acids, especially essential amino acids, can stimulate protein synthesis and muscle ana-bolism. What protein is best? The key is a combination of proteins that are more slowly released during the night. This means a mixture of whey pro-tein isolate, calcium caseinate, and milk protein isolate.

Whey protein isolate is important because it contains around 25 per-cent of the BCAAs (branched chain amino acids) leucine, isoleucine, and valine, and 50 percent essential amino acids. BCAAs have been clinically proven to inhibit muscle breakdown, especially in response to exercise—this can increase the net protein turnover during sleep and mean greater gains in lean muscle mass and better exercise recovery. Quality whey pro-tein isolate also provides key microfractions (tiny nutrients, such as lacto-ferrin, alpha-lactalbumin, and sialic acid), which have many positive effects in the body and can boost immune function—important in pre-bedtime nutrition (when the body is in a recovery state). If the immune system is not working at full strength, recovery during sleep may be hampered by excess free radicals and other damaging compounds.

Calcium caseinate is a more slowly released protein, providing amino acids to the body over a longer period of time. It has a high amount of L-glu-tamine, especially in the more easily absorbed peptide form. Glutamine is essential for increasing the rate of protein synthesis while reducing break-down in muscle tissue. Milk protein isolate contains both whey and casein. Taking 20–40 g (depending on body weight) of a high-quality whey isolate and calcium caseinate blend (mixed with water) about one to one-and-a-half hours before bedtime can do wonders for protein synthesis during sleep.

You may have heard that you should wake up in the middle of the night and drink a protein shake to keep the body in an anabolic state. How-ever, it is more important for optimal muscle building to not disturb sleep. Only if you get up due to some specific circumstance should you take a smaller amount (10–20 g) of a mixed protein drink to maximize absorption and minimize conversion to fat.

Pre-Bedtime Supplement Strategy

- **Growth hormone–releasing peptides (GHRPs)**—These oligopeptides have been shown to stimulate GH release. If you can afford them (they're somewhat expensive), they are worth trying, especially if you are over forty years of age. Take them one hour before bedtime on an empty stomach. Quality products in this category include GH STAK by Muscle-Link and Secretagogue-One by MHP.

- **L-Arginine**—Arginine helps boost nitric oxide levels, which leads to greater blood flow and nutrient transport. Arginine can help support protein synthesis as well. High doses of arginine seem to work better, upward of 5–10 grams before bedtime (however, this may cause stomach discomfort in some people).

- **Alpha GPC**—Short for L-alpha-glycerylphosphorylcholine, Alpha GPC is an acetylcholine precursor derived from soy. Small amounts (150–400 mg) seem to boost GH levels, which makes it cost-effective. It is available as a supplement ingredient in several products, including Kick Start from EAS.

- **Melatonin**—This is a natural hormone produced by the pineal gland. Research indicates that it may intensify REM sleep and, according to one study, it can boost GH levels, so taking it before bedtime can have a dual purpose. A dose of 2–5 mg before sleep may be helpful.

- **ZMA**—This is a special combination of zinc, magnesium, and vitamin B_6 that has been found to impact athletic performance and boost testosterone levels naturally. ZMA HP by EAS and ZMA by BioTest are quality ZMA products. Take the recommended dose thirty to forty-five minutes before bedtime.

- *Tribulus terrestris*—This herb, also known as puncture vine, has been shown to boost testosterone levels naturally. (It stimulates leutinizing hormone production from the pituitary gland, which in turn stimulates testosterone.) Taking 500–1,000 mg about thirty to forty-five minutes before bedtime can be beneficial. Quality tribulus products include Forza-T by Instone Nutrition and Tribex-500 by BioTest.

- **Phosphatidylserine (PS)**—PS is a phospholipid (a type of fat containing the mineral phosphorus and found in every cell) that is derived mainly from soy lecithin. Research has shown that PS may be a powerful cortisol-suppressing agent. Taking 400 mg about thirty minutes before bedtime can make a significant difference in recovery. A quality PS product is Cort-Bloc from Muscle-Link.

- **L-Glutamine** (preferably the more easily absorbed glutamine peptide)—This is one of the most important pre-bedtime supplements. Glutamine is the most abundant amino acid found in human muscle and plasma. In fact, 60 percent of the free-floating amino acid pool in skeletal muscle cells is made up of glutamine. It has come to be known as a "conditionally essential" amino acid because, in times of stress (including exercise), the body requires more of it to maintain both blood and muscle stores. Glutamine has tremendous benefits to exercising individuals and those looking to increase lean muscle mass and decrease body fat. It may also improve immune function and has been shown to boost GH levels in smaller doses. Many of these powerful effects can help increase lean body mass and reduce the breakdown of hard-earned muscle. Take 2–10 g (depending on body weight and training intensity) of glutamine thirty to forty-five minutes before bedtime. Quality glutamine supplements include Cytovol by EAS and Effervescent Glutamine by MHP.

- **Multivitamin/mineral and antioxidants**—These are key micronutrients that help regulate many reactions and processes in the body; individuals who exercise have a higher requirement for vitamins and minerals. Consider these a safety net that can help maximize the process of protein synthesis and muscle repair. Taking a good multivitamin/mineral formula before bed can really make a difference in recovery. Antioxidants are important because they can boost immune function and scavenge free radicals—exercise seems to enhance free radical production and antioxidants can neutralize them. Free radicals may also increase muscle soreness. One study showed that taking vitamin C (2 g) reduced oxidative stress and significantly enhanced recovery (again, a lot of recovery occurs at night while sleeping). Some quality multivitamin/mineral products include Opti-Pack by Super Nutrition and Mega Men by GNC. Take the recommended dose with your nightly protein shake and another dose with breakfast.

- **Water**—Being well hydrated before bed can allow the supplements you take to work more effectively. Don't drink too much water before bed as you will be racing to the bathroom all night—6–8 ounces of water about fifteen minutes prior to bed should be sufficient.

MEAL-REPLACEMENT POWDERS (MRPs)

If you fail to plan, then you plan to fail. Convenience can be a very important part of sticking to the Six-Pack Diet Plan and you will find meal-replacement powders (MRPs) to be quite convenient.

When following this program, it is important to eat six to eight small meals daily to increase nutrient absorption, enhance metabolic rate, and help stabilize blood sugar (and insulin) levels. As mentioned earlier, according to clinical research, eating small meals throughout the day has been shown to be beneficial.

Realistically, no one has the time to cook six to eight meals daily, so MRPs allow you to get some of your meals in a convenient and generally tasty manner. MRPs help improve overall nutrition and give you the key nutrients your body needs to improve health and physical performance.

Another great benefit to these products is they allow you to quantify exactly what you are consuming in terms or calories, protein, carbohydrates, and fat. This is important because daily caloric intake and the types of macronutrients consumed can go a long way in determining whether fat loss and lean muscle gain will be achieved. Unless you have a food scale and calorie count book with you wherever you go, it is hard to measure these quantities with whole foods.

However, whole foods should still be the predominant source of nutrition on this diet as they provide fiber (usually low in MRPs) and phytochemicals (plant chemicals from fruits and vegetables) vital to health. Plus, going a period of time relying solely on MRPs and without whole foods can decrease digestive enzyme activity, which is harmful for overall gastrointestinal function.

MRPs can be considered a complete meal as they usually contain protein, carbohydrates, fats, and vitamins and minerals. So-called low-carbohydrate MRPs are showing up on the market, but in many cases these are just protein powders in packets. There are also "light" versions of some MRPs, but the important thing is to get sufficient amounts of the macro - nutrients.

MRPs usually start with a "proprietary protein blend," as manufacturers have been in a "protein race" for some time. First there were 37 g of protein per serving, then 42 g, 45 g, 50 g, now 60 g—what's next? Contrary to some opinions, no research has shown that the body can only absorb a certain amount of protein at one time. Protein absorption depends on many factors, including metabolism, body weight, and exercise intensity but the body can absorb large amounts of protein in one sitting. Some MRPs may have only one protein source, such as whey protein isolate, but it is preferable to get a protein blend in order to utilize all the functional benefits of different proteins.

Listed below are some of the protein sources found in MRPs:

- Quality whey protein has many benefits, including providing intact immunoglobulins to support immune function, the highest concentration of BCAAs for the muscle-building process, a high biological value (readily absorbed and utilized by human muscle tissue), and the ability to dissolve well in liquid.

- Casein is a milk protein that seems to have a timed-release effect to slow the transit time of amino acids, which may enhance their absorption. It has a high natural glutamine content and most of this glutamine is found in the peptide form for better absorption. In one study, the ability of whey protein to build lean muscle mass, strength, and to lower body fat was compared with a casein protein hydrolysate and a hypocaloric (lower-calorie) diet. The results showed that those who used the casein protein group lost more body fat, gained more lean muscle mass, and had greater strength increases.

- Milk protein isolate contains both whey and casein and is a good source for these two proteins.

- Soy protein isolate has been shown to enhance thyroid hormone output, which can increase metabolic rate to support fat loss. It contains an excellent ratio of glutamine, arginine, and the BCAAs.

- Egg albumin protein boasts a great amino acid profile, but otherwise does not offer very many functional benefits. It is also a little harder to mix in liquid. The proteins in most MRPs are "agglomerated" or instantized, which means they go through a process that makes them easier to mix in liquid, making a blender unnecessary.

MRPs contain carbohydrates as well. Typically the main source is maltodextrin, which is a very low-cost ingredient derived from corn. Although it is considered a complex carbohydrate, it has a very high glycemic index rating. That means it can cause a large insulin response, which would be beneficial after a weight-training workout but not at other times of the day (although the protein in MRPs help balance out the blood sugar response). Another carbohydrate you'll see on MRP labels is corn syrup solids, which is also high glycemic. Fructose is fruit sugar and is added to MRPs not only to provide a source of carbohydrates, but also to sweeten the product; it is mainly metabolized in the liver. Brown rice syrup and brown rice complex are sometimes added to provide a good source of carbohydrates. Fructooligosaccharides (FOS) are derived from inulin and naturally found in Jerusalem artichokes—they can enhance the function of the digestive tract and also sweeten the product.

Some MRPs are fortified with dietary fiber, but many MRPs do not have a lot of fiber in them. Fiber makes an MRP thicker when mixed in water or juice.

Essential fatty acids (EFAs) are also added to MRPs, including borage oil, sunflower oil, flax seeds and flaxseed oil, MCTs (medium chain triglycerides, which are listed as saturated fats on the label but act differently than do saturated fats in the body), and primrose oil.

EFAs have many benefits including boosting metabolism; improving insulin action; increasing growth hormone and testosterone production; enhancing liver support and protection (especially borage oil and evening primrose oil); improving nerve function and energy production; and increasing nitrogen retention. Conjugated linoleic acid (CLA) is also showing up now in some MRPs. CLA is a "special fat" that helps with fat reduction and lean muscle mass gain. A lot of MRPs on the market that tout their low- or no-fat formulas are missing out on the benefits of EFAs.

MRPs contain a blend of vitamins and minerals to support overall health. Vitamins and minerals are usually ancillary items to MRPs and many minerals in the formulas, like calcium and magnesium, actually compete for absorption, and are usually not found in the more absorbable chelated forms. Chromium (usually in the polynicotinate form) is added to MRPs to support optimal blood sugar levels and help aid in fat loss. Also, many MRPs are higher in sodium, which may cause water retention to occur. It is good to look for an MRP that has at least a 2:1, or better yet 3:1 ratio of potassium-to-sodium to optimize water balance.

MRPs may have a lot of unnecessary ingredients, including artificial colors (to make the product look palatable), hydrogenated oils, and salt. MRPs are also sweetened with many different natural and artificial sweeteners, including sucralose, acesulfame K, aspartame, stevia, and kiwi extract. Most of these sweeteners are calorie free or contain calories in such a small amount as to be insignificant. Sucralose, a newcomer to the U.S. market, is 600 times sweeter than sugar; it has been tested in over 100 studies that confirm its safety and efficacy.

Aspartame seems to be controversial, as over 50 percent of the complaints the Food and Drug Administration (FDA) receives about food ingredients are related to aspartame. It is made of the amino acids phenylalanine and aspartic acid along with methanol (wood alcohol). There is plenty of safety data behind it, but many people seem to be sensitive to this sweetener. Individuals with phenylketonuria (PKU, a disorder in which the individual cannot metabolize phenylalanine), pregnant women, and nursing women should avoid aspartame.

Usage: Taking one to three MRP packets daily to effectively replace meals can be beneficial as part of the Six-Pack Diet Plan. The best times to take these products are after a workout or first thing in the morning as a breakfast replacement. Fresh (or frozen) fruit can be added, but keep in mind that you are also adding extra calories. If you are looking to lose fat, then mix MRPs with water, preferably cold water (adding ice may also help to improve the taste).

PROTEIN BARS

Protein bars usually contain protein, carbohydrates, fat, vitamins and minerals, and additional functional ingredients. Low-carbohydrate/high-protein bars are good for people looking to maintain lean muscle mass and lose body fat as part of the Six-Pack Diet Plan (although I do not advocate the use of protein bars when trying to get "super ripped"). These protein bars should contain good levels of the proteins recommended earlier in this chapter.

Corn syrup, high-fructose corn syrup (dextrose), rice syrup, maltitol, honey (invert sugar), turbinado sugar, sucrose, crisp rice, and fructose are all used as carbohydrate sources in bars. Fructose is fruit sugar added to bars to provide carbohydrates and to sweeten the product. It is mainly metabolized in the liver and therefore has a lower glycemic index. But consuming high amounts of fructose can lower metabolic rate and cause fat storage to occur, since the liver can metabolize only a certain amount of fructose.

Many people are concerned about the levels of carbohydrates in protein bars. This question has not only been raised by consumers but also by the FDA, which has now forced manufacturers to label glycerol and other sugar alcohols in protein bars as carbohydrates, even though they do not act like carbs in the body. That is why the carbohydrate content shot up drastically on the nutritional labels of protein bars. Of course, you'll also see terms like "net impact" carbs or "unavailable" carbs on the label as well, with some sort of fancy chart explaining it all. Manufacturers list these carbs separately to educate consumers that these nutrients have little or no impact on blood sugar levels.

Glycerol (also known as glycerin or glycerine) is a colorless, odorless, sweet-tasting nutrient. It is technically a trihydroxy alcohol found naturally as the backbone of triglycerides in the body. It is added to bars to help make them moist and to sweeten them. When taken in a protein bar, it does not cause any significant blood sugar response and seems to be eliminated from the body mostly unused. Glycerol has been shown to enhance athletic performance and cause "hyperhydration" when consumed with water (that is, it increases hydration levels above and beyond those levels achieved by ingesting water alone). It also seems to help keep the body cooler during exercise. Keep in mind that glycerol does contain 4.32 calories per gram.

It is very important to drink at least twelve to sixteen ounces of water with protein bars that contain glycerol in order to help lower the stomach discomfort sometimes associated with these bars and to maximize the hydration effects. In fact, when glycerol is ingested without water, it can actually cause dehydration. Also, eating too many glycerol-laden protein bars can cause water retention and bloating in some people.

A low-quality ingredient popping up in some protein bars is hydrolyzed collagen protein, also known as gelatin. This is an incomplete protein that is really cheap. If this protein is in the protein blend of a bar, I would be cautious about using it, especially if it's one of the main sources of protein. Hydrolyzed collagen does have some benefits in terms of joint and skin health, but not much for building quality muscle.

Protein bars also contain fat, including partially hydrogenated oils, fractionated vegetable oils, palm kernel oil, and peanut butter. A few bars have added essential fatty acids (EFAs), but it is very difficult to preserve EFA quality due to their sensitivity to light, heat, and oxygen. Most of the fat (especially the saturated fat) found in bars is in the chocolate coating. Saturated fats have been linked to many health problems including cardiovascular disease. Partially hydrogenated oils are trans fatty acids produced during the hydrogenation process. Hydrogenated oils increase the shelf-life of products, but they are very detrimental to health and may increase cholesterol and interfere with the liver's detoxification system. Fractionated oils seem to be healthier for you. Fractionation is the separating of oil into two or more triglyceride fractions with different chemical properties. In other words, it allows weaker oils to be changed into better oils.

The basic bar-making process from a quality manufacturer goes like this: the main ingredients (including the proteins) are mixed together (manually or using an industrial-sized mixer) with water, then the mixture is laid on a table evenly and goes through a machine process (the cooling tunnel/extruder) where it is cooled. Next, the bar is taken out of the cooling machine and coated with chocolate (enrobed). Finally, the bar sheets are cut and packaged.

Most high-protein bars on the market are not baked nowadays, so if the raw materials are high quality, then the protein microfractions stay intact. However, the raw ingredients may be subjected to heat. Manufacturers can provide you with certificates of analysis for the proteins in the bar (and for the bar itself), which will provide information about the quality of the protein you are getting. Some granola-type bars and those that contain rolled oats are baked and the proteins in them lose the microfractions in the baking process.

Usage: As a meal replacement or between-meal protein boost, consume one to two bars daily. Drink at least twelve to sixteen ounces of water with each bar. If you have stomach discomfort, eating the bars very slowly and drinking plenty of water can help.

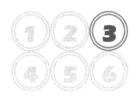

Fat-Loss
Supplements

ONE OF THE KEYS TO LOSING FAT QUICKLY and keeping it off permanently is the use of natural supplements. Research has demonstrated that a number of nutrients can help boost the body's ability to burn off fat. Thermogenic nutrients contain stimulating substances that increase metabolism so that normal body processes use up more calories. For those who may be sensitive to stimulants, there are also a number of non-stimulant nutrients that can help you lose more fat. These supplements play a vital role in the Six-Pack Diet Plan.

THERMOGENIC SUPPLEMENTS

Thermogenic nutrients boost body metabolism so that you can naturally burn more calories. Thermogenic supplements are booming because everyone is looking to shed those extra pounds. In this chapter, we'll investigate these thermogenic weight-loss ingredients and shed some light on their efficacy.

Citrus aurantium

Citrus aurantium (bitter orange or zhi shi) is an herb that contains the active ingredient synephrine as well as other potent compounds, such as octopamine and tyramine. It is touted as an ephedra alternative, now that ephedra has been demonized and banned. Think of it as ephedra's calmer chemical cousin, which means it still has thermogenic (fat-burning) effects while being less stimulating to the central nervous system. A study in *Current Therapeutic Research* showed that a combination of *Citrus aurantium* extract, caffeine, and St. John's wort caused significant body fat loss in overweight, healthy adults. Other research has looked at the thermogenic properties of compounds found in *Citrus aurantium,* including synephrine and octopamine, and the results are very promising.

Dosage: An efficacious dose is 20 milligrams (mg) of active standardized synephrine two to three times daily. (Do not take it if you are sensitive to stimulants or have any medical conditions.)

Caffeine

Caffeine (chemically, a methylxanthine) is one of the best-researched ergogenic aids (physical performance enhancers) available. Caffeine promotes fat oxidation and both weight and fat loss in exercising individuals. Many studies show that caffeine enhances both short- and long-term endurance performance. Caffeine seems to delay fatigue (prolonging time to exhaustion), so aerobic workouts can continue for longer periods. One study, published in the *International Journal of Sports Medicine* in 1998, states that "caffeine ingestion can be an effective ergogenic aid for short-term, supramaximal [full speed] running performance." Even though there are far fewer studies with caffeine and resistance training (weight lifting), some evidence suggests that caffeine can increase the power generated in repeated muscle contractions and enhance endurance at submaximal (about 75 percent full strength) tension.

Caffeine works through several mechanisms of action, including promoting the use of stored fat for energy; releasing calcium from the sarcoplasmic reticulum—a part of the cell from which calcium is released—(thereby leading to greater muscle contraction and force production); antagonism of the adenosine receptors in the central nervous system (which can help enhance focus and mental function); and inhibition of phosphodiesterases (leading to an increase of cyclic andenosine monophosphate (AMP) in muscle tissue thus creating a more favorable intracellular environment in active muscle). Caffeine also spares glycogen (carbohydrate stores in muscle cells and the liver) leading to an increased rate of fat oxidation, which could explain why caffeine delays time to exhaustion during aerobic exercise. Caffeine has some diuretic properties that can aid in decreasing water retention in the body, although it does not seem to act as a diuretic during exercise. Nevertheless, it is important to consume plenty of water when taking caffeine.

One thing to be cautious about is caffeine's effects on blood sugar.

Although not clear from the research, it may decrease insulin sensitivity, so diabetics need to be careful. Regularly consuming high doses may also adversely affect blood pressure. Moderation is the key to ingesting caffeine. A regular cup of coffee has about 100 mg of caffeine per serving, but some research shows that pure caffeine (in pill, powder or liquid form) may be more effective than coffee in maximizing caffeine's benefits. A combination of guarana and yerba mate (and damiana leaf) was actually shown in a study published in the *Journal of Human Nutrition and Dietetics* to significantly enhance weight loss after just forty-five days of use.

Dosage: Take 200 mg of caffeine forty-five minutes before a workout.

Green Tea Extract

Green tea has been widely used for its immuno-enhancing effects and anti-cancer properties. The major components of interest in green tea extract are polyphenols, including epigallocatechin gallate (EGCG) and caffeine. Research shows that this potent extract provides greater antioxidant protection than vitamins C and E.

What many people don't know is that green tea extract may have great potential as a fat burner. A study published in the *American Journal of Clinical Nutrition* showed that it actually increased twenty-four-hour energy expenditure and fat oxidation in humans. This may be due to its caffeine content, since caffeine also has some of these properties, but the authors of this study concluded that "green tea extract has thermogenic properties and promotes fat oxidation beyond that explained by its caffeine content per se. Green tea extract may play a role in the control of body composition via sympathetic activation of thermogenesis, fat oxidation, or both."

Its effectiveness is most likely linked to its EGCG content. Another recent study showed that the synergy of green tea's catechin polyphenol and caffeine ingredients stimulates brown adipose tissue thermogenesis. Green tea extract, and the synergistic relationship of its components, may be a valuable tool in the management of obesity.

Dosage: Taking 200–300 mg of green tea extract daily could be beneficial; look for a standardized extract containing at least 40 percent EGCG.

Coleus forskohlii

Although not a stimulant ingredient, *Coleus forskohlii* is showing up in many thermogenic weight-loss formulas. *Coleus forskohlii* (active ingredient, forskolin) is a "power" herb that increases the amount of cyclic AMP (adenosine monophosphate) in cells. Increasing cyclic AMP (cAMP) levels provides several benefits for athletes, including relaxing the arteries and smooth muscles; lowering blood pressure; enhancing insulin secretion (which can help drive carbohydrates and protein into muscle cells for energy and recovery); increasing thyroid hormone function (to help enhance metabolic rate); and significantly increasing lipolysis (fat burning). In addition to enhancing lipolysis, Forskolin may also inhibit fat storage.

Dosage: A typical dose is 100 mg *Coleus forskohlii,* standardized to 20 percent forskolin, or take 25–60 mg of forskolin daily in three divided doses. The Sabinsa Corporation has a quality product called ForsLean®.

Cayenne Pepper

Cayenne pepper has been known for hundreds of years to increase perspiration and influence body temperature. Cayenne has unique metabolic and thermogenic properties based on its capsaicin content (the active ingredient). Its effects on thermogenesis are mainly attributed to capsaicin's activation of the sympathetic nervous system (stimulation of the hormones epinephrine and norepinephrine). This results in enhanced energy metabolism, more calories burned, and a feeling of warmth. According to research, cayenne pepper can also help decrease appetite and lower food intake. When looking for a cayenne pepper product, make sure it contains a standardized amount of capsaicin (0.25% of extract).

Dosage: Typically 30 mg of cayenne three times daily. You can also sprinkle cayenne pepper on each of your food meals to really fire things up!

Bioperine®

Bioperine is derived from black pepper, a spice found in the kitchen cupboards of most households. The compound piperine comes from an extract of the small pepper berry. Piperine has been shown to significantly enhance the absorption of various nutrients, while generating an increase in metabolic action to help support fat loss. Some of the clinical trials with Bioperine (provided from the Sabinsa Corporation) showed it is a "natural thermonutrient and bioavailability enhancer." As a thermonutrient, Bioperine has a thermogenic effect on the body's metabolic rate: the higher the metabolic rate, the more heat produced by the body, thereby enhancing the fat-burning process.

Dosage: A typical dose is 5 mg of Bioperine taken one to three times daily, preferably with other fat-loss nutrients.

Naringin

Naringin, a flavonoid compound found in grapefruit, gives grapefruit its characteristic bitter flavor. This ingredient appears in some fat-loss formulas, mainly to increase the effects of caffeine in these products. It can increase the half-life of some supplements (thereby lowering the rate at which the supplement clears the body). It does this by interfering with enzymatic activity in the intestines. One caution is to avoid this ingredient with prescription medicines as it can prolong their effects as well.

Dosage: Typically take 100 mg of naringin two to three times daily with caffeine-containing products.

L-Tyrosine

The amino acid tyrosine acts as a direct precursor to the neurotransmitters dopamine, norepinephrine, and epinephrine. It seems to work synergistically with thermogenic supplements that include ephedrine/synephrine and caffeine. This amino acid has been called the "focus" supplement because it enhances mental focus and mental clarity, which is especially useful before a workout. It seems to delay mental fatigue and boosts exercise performance by lowering neurotransmitter "burnout." Some recent research confirms the performance-enhancing effects of tyrosine in exercise. Interestingly, tyrosine also helps manufacture thyroid hormones, which regulate metabolism in the body.

Dosage: Efficacious doses range from 1–3 grams (g) daily in two divided doses. Taking tyrosine one hour before training can help boost exercise performance.

Quality thermogenic products that contain many of the nutrients discussed above include Lean Fire from Instone Nutrition, Lean System 7 from iSatori Global Technologies, and Hydroxycut from MuscleTech. For an additional boost, take the recommended dose forty-five minutes before training, especially before cardiovascular work, with plenty of water. You can use these products during phases 1 and 2 of the Six-Pack Diet Plan (for a duration of twelve weeks) and then take a few months off during the maintenance phase. (See Putting It All Together for more details.)

Non-Stimulant Supplements

Recently, a new category of fat-loss products has emerged that claims to help you burn fat without stimulants. There was definitely a need for these products as many people were either getting "burned out" using thermogenic supplements or were actually sensitive to some of the ingredients in thermogenic fat burners, such as caffeine. Non-stimulant fat burners can still be quite stimulating in terms of fat loss. For those people who do not have a problem using stimulant supplements, these non-stimulant products can actually be combined with them to further promote fat burning—just watch out for any doubling up of ingredients. Keep in mind that only some of the following supplements have adequate research validation at this time.

Guggulsterones

To begin the discussion about guggulsterones (guggulipid), we must first talk about thyroid hormones. Thyroid hormones are very important for normal growth and development and they maintain metabolic stability by regulating oxygen requirements, body weight, and intermediary metabolism (enzyme-driven processes within cells that extract energy from nutrient molecules and use that energy to construct cellular components). They exert effects on thermogenesis and temperature regulation and can enhance lipolysis (fat burning) in fat tissue.

Guggulipid is a staple in Ayruvedic medicine, a holistic approach to health care practiced in India for centuries. It is derived from the plant *Commiphora mukul*. There have been several research studies done with this herb that show very positive benefits. One study published in *The Journal of the Association of Physicians in India* showed that guggulipid had a strong effect in decreasing triglycerides (fats) as well as LDL ("bad" cholesterol) levels, while increasing HDL ("good" cholesterol) levels in humans. It has these functional effects because it may cause an increase in thyroid hormones (both T4 and T3). There are several other studies that have shown similar effects of guggulipid as a fat-reducing compound. This natural compound has also been shown to be safe and completely nontoxic in humans.

Dosage: A typical dose is 25 mg active guggulsterones (after standardization) taken three times daily. One dose with plenty of water thirty minutes before cardiovascular exercise can be helpful. When choosing a guggulipid product, make sure it is a standardized guggulsterone of type E and Z from the plant *Commiphora mukul*. Good pure guggul supplements include T3 by SAN and Guggulbolic by Syntrax.

7-Keto DHEA

DHEA (dehydroepiandrosterone) is a natural hormone produced by the adrenal glands that is a precursor to other hormones. The metabolite 7-keto DHEA does not convert into the sex steroids, testosterone and estrogen, so it can provide many of the benefits of DHEA, such as increased energy, sex drive, and even fat loss, without any unwanted side effects. In fact, several studies show that this compound can have powerful fat-burning effects in healthy individuals. One study in *Current Therapeutic Research* showed that 7-keto DHEA caused three times more fat loss versus a placebo. According to the research, 7-keto DHEA may increase levels of the thyroid hormone T3, which can lead to increased metabolism and greater fat burning.

Dosage: A typical dose is 100 mg of 7-keto DHEA taken one to two times daily. Good sources of 7-keto DHEA are Lean System 7 by iSatori Global Technologies or Lean Fire from Instone Nutrition.

Phosphates

Phosphates are compounds that contain the mineral phosphorus and may help boost metabolism and possibly exercise performance. For instance, potassium phosphate may enhance recovery after exercise. Phosphates may also delay fatigue by buffering lactic acid and they can help store creatine more efficiently in muscle cells (as creatine phosphate). According to a study in the *Journal of Physiology and Pharmacology*, a combination of calcium, potassium, and sodium phosphates was shown to increase resting metabolic rate in overweight women who were on a low-calorie diet. The authors of this study concluded that phosphates may play a role in the peripheral metabolism of thyroid hormones specifically by preventing a decrease in T3 output. Another study showed that calcium and potassium phosphate supplementation is useful in increasing metabolic rate and helping with fat loss.

Dosage: A typical dose is 1 g of phosphates taken one hour prior to exercise. Some people may experience stomach discomfort with this dose, so a lower dose may be used to allow the body to adapt. A good product to try is Phosphate Edge by FSI Nutrition.

Theobromine

Theobromine is a natural compound found in cocoa and chocolate. It is a member of the methylxanthine family (similar to caffeine), but is a very mild stimulant that can have an energizing effect on the body. It may also enhance metabolic rate and improve the feeling of well-being (as many chocolate lovers have experienced). Theobromine is a mild diuretic (increases urine production) and relaxes the smooth muscles of the bronchi in the lungs. Very few side effects have been reported with theobromine ingestion.

Dosage: A typical recommended dosage is 400 mg of theobromine taken two to three times daily.

Conjugated Linoleic Acid

Conjugated linoleic acid (CLA) has been shown in recent studies to have profound fat-loss effects in humans. It can lower abdominal fat and is thus a key nutrient in the Six-Pack Diet Plan. This advanced form of an essential fatty acid can actually reduce body fat while dieting. It is naturally found in beef and dairy products, but supplementation is the only way to get effi-cacious doses. Research indicates that CLA can help increase lean body mass and act as an antioxidant as well.

Researchers have proposed several mechanisms by which CLA works. It may interfere with a substance in your body called lipoprotein lipase that helps store fat. CLA also helps your body use its existing fat for energy. So, you prevent fat storage while burning the fat you already have. Recent long-term research on CLA showed that it caused a significant decrease in body fat while increasing lean body mass. Taking CLA supplementation for a year caused a 9 percent reduction in body fat and a 2 percent increase in lean muscle mass. Another study conducted at Maastricht University in the Netherlands indicated that CLA may support the building of fat-free mass after weight loss. This study also showed that CLA supplementation at a dose of either 1.8 g/daily or 3.6 g/daily caused an increase in resting meta-bolic rate and revving up the metabolism can result in greater fat loss.

One interesting application of CLA is blood sugar regulation. A study published in the *Journal of Nutrition* showed that CLA had positive effects on fasting blood sugar levels and may have some potential in treating dia-betes. The researchers even theorized that CLA could have an effect on appetite due to its modification of the hormone leptin.

Dosage: Effective doses range from 1.4 to 4.0 g of CLA daily. However, watch out for "nighttime liquid" formulas, weight-loss bars, and other products that contain low amounts (less than 1 g daily) of CLA, which may not have any effect.

Hydroxycitric Acid

Hydroxycitric acid (HCA) or hydroxycitrate is the main acid derived from the fruit of the *Garcinia cambogia* tree, found mainly in Southeast Asia. This is certainly not a new or little-known ingredient; in fact, it has been studied quite extensively for years. HCA acts as an appetite suppressant through the enhancement of serotonin levels (by stimulating its release and inhibiting its re-uptake). Increasing serotonin levels has been shown to decrease food intake, enhance mood, and lower weight gain. Controlling food intake is a key determining factor for losing fat.

Human studies with HCA have been equivocal, showing mostly mixed results. Several studies show no effect on weight loss while other studies show good effects using HCA. One fairly large, well-controlled study on HCA, published in the *Journal of the American Medical Association,* concluded that "*Garcinia cambogia* failed to produce significant weight loss and fat mass loss beyond that observed with placebo." This study used a low dose (1,500 mg daily) of HCA and the subjects in the study were on a low-calorie diet. These may be reasons why the HCA did not produce significant results. Other studies on HCA using a similar dose have shown no significant effects either. Higher doses seem to be necessary to have an effect on weight/fat loss.

However, a study at Georgetown University Medical Center showed much better results with HCA supplementation. Individuals using HCA for eight weeks lost a significant amount of weight, lowered their total cholesterol, raised their HDL (good) cholesterol, and experienced appetite suppression through increased serotonin levels. The HCA used in this study was a more potent extract called Super CitriMax. The dosage and timing of ingestion is the key with HCA: this study, for example, used 2,800 mg of HCA daily, in three divided doses taken thirty minutes before meals.

Another recent study suggests lower doses of HCA may be useful for appetite suppression. This study showed that 300 mg of HCA taken three times daily reduced energy intake while sustaining satiety (the ability to eat less but still feel satisfied).

A good HCA supplement is CitriMax from Optibolic (available at GNC stores and elsewhere). HCA can also be found in Hydroxycut from Muscle-Tech. Unfortunately, many companies put low doses of HCA in their products and claim weight-loss benefits. Make sure that any product you purchase contains the right (efficacious) dose of HCA.

Dosage: HCA should be taken thirty minutes before meals three times daily for at least four weeks. An efficacious dose for weight loss is 2,500 to 3,000 mg daily of active HCA (after standardization from *Garcinia cambogia*). For appetite suppression, lower doses may be helpful. HCA seems to be very safe, with no side effects reported in the majority of studies.

L-Carnitine

Carnitine is a vitamin-like compound that may enhance fat utilization when taken prior to exercise, although research on this nutrient has been equivocal. L-carnitine works by promoting the transport and metabolism of long-chain fatty acids into the mitochondria to be used for energy. It is a naturally occurring compound found in meats and dairy products, so vegetarians may benefit most from supplementation. L-carnitine has been shown to have effects that benefit the heart as well. Some research suggests that it may enhance endurance (since fat is the major metabolic fuel for long-term aerobic exercise).

In terms of weight loss, a fairly high dose (2 g twice daily) was shown to have no effect on fat loss when combined with light exercise in overweight women. The problem may be getting carnitine into muscle tissues. This supplement may have some uses, but it certainly has not lived up to its weight-loss hype. Many products on the market contain low doses of carnitine just to claim that they have it. There is some new research that shows that L-carnitine L-tartrate (a special form of L-carnitine) can actually assist significantly in recovery from hard training. This may prove to be one of its best uses.

Dosage: I wouldn't recommend carnitine for fat loss until more comprehensive research is done, but for exercise recovery, taking 1–2 grams one hour before training can be helpful. Liquid L-carnitine supplements may be better absorbed. However, watch out for low, ineffective doses in some products (less than 500 mg).

Dandelion Root (*Taraxacum officinale*)

Although not necessarily a fat burner per se, dandelion root is showing up in many non-stimulant fat-loss formulas. This is because it helps lower water retention—holding water can make you look bloated. Dandelion root has been shown to act as a natural diuretic without causing a mineral imbalance or potassium depletion like some diuretic drugs. It can also have beneficial effects on the liver. Dandelion contains high levels of vitamin A and choline.

Dosage: Typically take 250–500 mg of dandelion root three times daily; look for a 4:1 standardized extract.

A product that contains many of the non-stimulant ingredients discussed above is AbGONE from BioTech Research; take two capsules three times daily with meals.

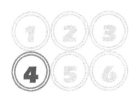

Hormone-Modifying Strategies

HORMONES CAN BE MAJOR ALLIES in your war on fat. There are various strategies and nutrients that can actually boost your own hormones naturally. By using these key nutrients and other options at appropriate times, you can be on your way to a lean and healthy physique.

MAXIMIZING GROWTH HORMONE LEVELS

Growth hormone (GH) increases lean body mass, reduces body fat, boosts energy, enhances immune function, and even improves sexual function. Obesity diminishes the release of GH and fasting actually helps increase it. Optimizing GH levels can help you get lean abs.

- Growth hormone (GH) levels seem to be high during a fasting state, so try not to eat one hour before bedtime to maximize its release during the fasting hours of sleep and to enhance the recovery process.

- Too much insulin seems to interfere with GH release, so avoid carbohydrates and pure whey protein before bedtime.

- Get at least seven to nine hours of sleep per night, without interruption, because this is the primary time for GH release.

- Weight train regularly, as this has been shown to help increase GH levels. This is due to the increase in protein synthesis that becomes necessary secondary to weight training. Biochemically, an increase in lactic acid production due to intense exercise leads to an increase in cyclic AMP (adenosine monophosphate), which then increases GH levels.

- Take growth hormone–releasing peptides (GHRPs)—These oligopeptides, also known as secretagogues, have been shown to stimulate GH release. A relatively new study confirms the benefits of these secretagogues taken along with exercise. However, more research needs to be done and these products are expensive. If you can afford them, they are worth trying, especially if you are over forty years old (since natural GH levels tend to decline after this age). Take GHRPs one hour before bedtime on an empty stomach. A quality product in this category is GH-Stak by Muscle-Link.

- Try L-arginine—This non-essential amino acid (sometimes considered "conditionally essential") has equivocal evidence that it can boost GH levels; some studies show little effect of L-arginine as a GH booster, while other studies show good results. High doses seem to work better, around 5–10 grams (g) before bedtime (however, this amount may cause stomach discomfort in some people).

- Take Alpha GPC—Short for L-alpha-glycerylphosphorylcholine, this is an acetylcholine precursor derived from soy that has been shown in preliminary research to boost GH levels and increase neurological function. Relatively small amounts of 150–400 milligrams (mg) seem to be effective.

BOOSTING TESTOSTERONE

Testosterone is called the most powerful muscle-building hormone because it does just that—builds muscle and boosts strength quickly. Testosterone increases muscle protein synthesis and net muscle protein balance, resulting in increased muscle mass. It also enhances sex drive and energy levels. By maximizing testosterone levels, you can enhance lean muscle mass, which can lead to increased metabolic rate and hence, fat loss.

- Eat plenty of essential fatty acids, especially monounsaturated fats, since they stimulate good prostaglandins, which are hormone-like substances that influence testosterone. Essential fatty acids can be found in natural peanut butter, flaxseed oil, olive oil, and canola oil. Eating fish regularly, including salmon, can also help.

- Perform compound exercises like the squat and bench press and try to use heavy weights for a lower number of reps. These exercises and training methods have been shown to boost testosterone levels more than other types of isolation exercises. See Chapter 6 for more information on weight training.

- Stop alcohol intake—Alcohol can reduce testosterone production.

- Don't eat too much protein—I know most weight trainers have been indoctrinated with the idea of eating huge amounts of protein, but research indicates that too much protein can lower testosterone levels. Eating 1–1.5 g of protein per pound of body weight daily is plenty. This is about the amount of protein that is recommended in the Six-Pack Diet Plan.

- Supplement with ZMA—This is a special combination of zinc, magnesium, and vitamin B_6 that has been found to impact athletic performance and boost testosterone levels. ZMA-T by Muscle-Link and ZMA by BioTest are both high-quality products. Take the recommended dose thirty to forty-five minutes before bedtime.

- Try *Tribulus terrestris*—This herb, also known as puncture vine, increases testosterone levels naturally. Taking 500–1,000 mg about thirty to forty-five minutes before bedtime or a workout can be beneficial. Quality tribulus products are Acetabolan-II by MuscleTech (this product also includes acetyl-L-carnitine, which may have some beneficial effects on testosterone levels) and Tribex 500 by BioTest.

ENHANCING THYROID HORMONES

Thyroid hormones maintain metabolism, body weight, and intermediary metabolism. Metabolism represents all the body processes that expend calories; intermediary metabolism is how those processes work together to boost energy expenditure, heat production, and more. Thyroid hormones influence thermogenesis and temperature regulation and can enhance lipolysis (fat burning) in adipose (fat) tissue. This is essential for getting six-pack abs and a lean body.

- Eat six to eight small meals throughout the day—One study published in the *Canadian Journal of Physiology and Pharmacology* showed that increased frequency of feeding helped stabilize insulin secretion and increased thermogenesis and fat utilization. Eating more frequently may help keep thyroid hormones working at optimal levels.

Hormone Testing Methods

To effectively use these hormone-modifying strategies, you need to know where you stand in terms of your hormones, so it is wise to have them tested a few times per year. If one or more of your hormones are deficient, then incorporate some of the tips in this chapter to help normalize levels. There are two accurate ways to measure hormone levels: blood and saliva tests.

Blood Tests—Blood is a more comprehensive (and expensive) way to test for hormones. The benefit is that you can test virtually anything using this method and it is more likely to be covered by insurance. However, it requires a visit to the doctor or a blood-testing center. This can be inconvenient and the blood may not be drawn at the right times for accurate measuring (for example, a morning cortisol measurement). Plus, you have to measure the "free" form of the hormone to get an accurate reading because the "bound" form can also show up, leading to a false reading. If you want to use this method, your doctor can routinely perform these blood tests. To do it yourself, try the Life Extension Foundation (www.lef.org) or go to one of their blood-drawing stations nationwide. (For more information, call 800-208-3444.) The recommended tests for both men and women include free testosterone, estradiol (a form of estrogen), morning cortisol, IGF-1, and free T3.

Saliva Tests—The benefits of saliva testing are convenience and lower cost. Plus, saliva hormones are in their "free" or active states, so this allows for an exact and accurate reading. Anyone can do saliva testing without having to go through his or her doctor (except in California and New York). The downside to saliva testing is that thyroid hormone and IGF-1 levels are not usually measurable with this method. Unfortunately, these tests are usually not covered by insurance. A good source for saliva tests is ZRT Laboratory in Oregon (www.salivatest.com). Tests for men and women include testosterone, estradiol, and morning cortisol. You can test other hormones as well, but these are the key ones for muscle building and fat loss.

- Have one high-calorie, "cheat" meal per week—This can help boost metabolism again during calorie restrictive eating. You can do this during the maintenance phase of the Six-Pack Diet Plan. (See Putting It All Together.)

- Take guggulsterones—Guggulsterones (also known as guggulipid) from the plant *Commiphora mukul* have been used for hundreds of years in Ayurvedic medicine. They can boost metabolism by increasing thyroid hormone levels (both T4 and T3). There are several studies that have shown the effects of guggulipid as a fat-reducing compound. An effective dose is 25 mg active guggulsterones (after standardization) taken three times daily. One good guggul supplement is T3 from SAN.

- Phosphates—Phosphates are mineral compounds that contain phosphorus and may help boost metabolism and possibly exercise performance. According to a study published in the *Journal of Physiology and Pharmacology,* a combination of calcium, potassium, and sodium phosphates were shown to increase resting metabolic rates in overweight women who were on a low-calorie diet. The authors of this study concluded that phosphates may play a role in the metabolism of thyroid hormones, specifically by preventing a decrease in T3 output. A typical dose is 1 g of phosphates taken one hour prior to exercise. One recommended product is Phosphate Edge by FSI Nutrition.

MASTERING INSULIN AND BLOOD SUGAR

Insulin is primarily responsible for the direction of energy metabolism after eating. It can help transport key nutrients like glucose and amino acids into muscle cells, but it can also cause fat storage to occur. It is important to control insulin levels and have this hormone working in your favor when trying to get lean.

- It is important to raise and lower insulin levels at different times of the day. For example, insulin sensitivity is high early in the morning and right after a workout. Knowing this, you can maximize the use of insulin to drive nutrients into muscle cells during these key times. Spiking insulin levels after a workout by consuming simple carbohydrates and protein (preferably in liquid form) can block the catabolic effects of the hormone cortisol and allow for key nutrients to replenish muscle cells. Nutrient uptake is very high after a workout due to enzymatic activity and higher insulin sensitivity. Spiking insulin levels can also enhance protein synthesis and lower the breakdown of protein secondary to weight training. Take a good high-carb/moderate-protein drink within fifteen to twenty minutes after a workout session. A 3:1 or 4:1 ratio of carbohydrates to proteins is recommended.

- There are also times when you want to lower insulin as much as possible to prevent fat storage from occurring. One of these key times is at night before bedtime. Spiking insulin levels near bedtime can actually decrease or even suppress GH levels, which can in turn lower the recovery process and impede muscle growth. Since metabolism is generally slower at night, eating carbohydrates or certain amino acids (the BCAAs leucine, isoleucine, and valine) can cause an insulin response and cause greater fat storage at this time. It is a good idea to lower carb intake at night and eat more fiber and protein. One secret to the Six-Pack Diet Plan is to eat only protein and fiber at night.

- Eat low-glycemic meals (foods that have a lesser impact on blood sugar levels)—Mixed meals containing high-quality protein, complex carbo- hydrates, and essential fats are the key to stabilizing insulin levels.

Supplements for Optimal Insulin and Blood Sugar Levels

Insulin can be a powerful ally in building muscle mass and reducing body fat. Controlling insulin and blood sugar levels can go a long way toward a great physique and getting fabulous "beach-worthy" abs. Since these sup- plements help stabilize blood sugar levels and support insulin release, it is a good idea to take them with carbohydrate-containing meals. Dosages will vary, so it is best to contact your physician to discuss correct doses based on your medical history.

Alpha-Lipoic Acid

Also known as lipoic acid or thioctic acid, alpha-lipoic acid is a sulfur-con- taining antioxidant produced naturally by the body and found in foods such as liver, brewer's yeast, and potatoes. Alpha-lipoic acid is a unique and powerful antioxidant and insulin mimicker, which plays a key role in pro- ducing cellular energy. It is actually prescribed in some parts of Europe for blood sugar disorders.

In the metabolic cycle, alpha-lipoic acid acts as a coenzyme in the pro- duction of energy by converting carbohydrates into energy (ATP). Carbo- hydrates are broken down into sugars, resulting in pyruvic acid, which in turn breaks down to an enzyme complex that contains alpha-lipoic acid. The end result is more energy. This action is important for people who exercise, since higher levels of energy may be desired, and often required. Alpha-lipoic acid is a necessary component of the energy transport reactions that allow for glucose to be metabolized into energy. It can also help your fitness efforts by normalizing blood sugar levels, while metabolizing sugar into energy.

Dosage: A typical dose is 100 mg taken three times daily with meals.

Chromium

Chromium is an essential trace element needed for normal protein, fat, and carbohydrate metabolism. It is important for energy production and also plays a key role in regulating appetite, reducing sugar cravings, and increasing lean body mass. Chromium helps insulin metabolize fat, turn protein into muscle, and convert sugar into energy. The primary function of chromium is to potentiate the effects of insulin and thereby enhance glucose, amino acid, and fat metabolism. It does this by enhancing insulin sensitivity.

Exercise induces chromium losses in athletes and may lead to chromium deficiency, resulting in impaired insulin function. The biologically active component of glucose tolerance factor (GTF), which potentiates insulin activity and is responsible for normal insulin function, is dependent on chromium. Due to the excessive chromium loss during vigorous exercise, athletes may have an increased requirement for chromium.

Chromium (particularly the polynicotinate or nicotinate form) has been shown to ameliorate type II diabetes, reduce hypertension, help decrease fat mass and increase lean body mass, and reduce weight.

Dosage: A great time to take chromium is after a weight-training session. Take 200–400 micrograms (mcg) to further enhance insulin sensitivity and improve nutrient transport. Taking 200 mcg three to four times daily, in addition to the post-workout dose, can also be useful.

Vanadyl Sulfate

Vanadyl sulfate is a form of the trace mineral vanadium, which is thought to help increase glucose transport into muscle cells. It may preferentially allow for glucose to be stored in muscle cells versus fat storage. It is considered an "insulin mimetic" (that is, mimics insulin), but the higher doses at which this property is found may be toxic to humans. Vanadium may have added potential as less toxic forms are discovered. Vanadyl sulfate also has poor bioavailability (blood and tissue absorption).

Vanadyl sulfate has been shown to support healthy blood sugar levels in type II diabetics and may increase insulin sensitivity up to four weeks after vanadium supplementation has ended. But just because an ingredient can mimic the effects of insulin, it may still have no effect on exercise performance. For example, a study published in the *International Journal of Sports Nutrition* showed that vanadyl sulfate supplementation had no significant effect on body composition or exercise performance in weight-training athletes. This nutrient has not lived up to its hype, but it may still be useful in some forms.

Dosage: A typical dose is 45 mg of vanadyl sulfate taken twice daily.

Gymnema sylvestre

Gymnema sylvestre is a woody, vine-like plant that has been used for centuries in Ayurvedic medicine. The medicinally active parts of the plant are the leaves and roots. Clinical tests show that regular use of gymnema over a period of three to four months helped to reduce glycosuria, the appearance of carbohydrates in urine; that is, it helps utilize carbohydrates for energy or glycogen production instead of fat storage. Recent clinical trials conducted in India have shown that an extract of *Gymnema sylvestre* is useful for controlling blood sugar.

Gymnema sylvestre has an active compound called gymnemic acid made up of molecules that are similar to glucose. Those molecules fill the receptor locations on the taste buds for a period of one to two hours, thereby preventing the taste buds from being activated by any sugar molecules present in food. This helps lower sugar absorption—so if you eat sugar, it helps neutralize it. Similarly, the glucose-like molecules in gymnemic acid fill the receptor locations in the absorptive layers of the intestine, thereby preventing absorption of sugar molecules. Due to the change in the absorption of sugar, there is a consequent change in the blood sugar level.

Dosage: The recommended dose is 150 mg (standardized to 75 percent gymnemic acids) taken three to four times daily with carbohydrate-containing meals (especially sugar).

Glucosol (Corosolic Acid)

Glucosol is derived from the plant *Lagerstroemia speciosa L.* (Banaba), which acts as a glucose transport stimulator. A glucose transporter is important in regulating the level of intracellular glucose, an important function of all cells for acquiring energy. Modifications of glucose transport may cause several physiological effects, such as lowering blood and intracellular glucose levels.

Only a few compounds, insulin, for example, have been known to affect glucose transport activity. Researchers at Hiroshima University School of Medicine, in Japan, have studied the beneficial effects of corosolic acid, the insulin-like principle in Glucosol, and found that it causes a hypoglycemic effect (low blood sugar level).

Glucosol is called phyto-insulin (an insulin-like principle) because of its ability to aid in blood sugar regulation. Because it mimics the actions of insulin, it may also aid in creatine transport into muscle tissue. This is important because it allows creatine to be much more effective in increasing energy levels and promoting lean muscle mass. This compound can also increase energy levels by elevating carbohydrate stores in the muscle (glycogen).

Dosage: For weight loss, take 16 mg of Glucosol (available from SoftGel Technologies) two to three times daily, one dose after a workout.

D-Pinitol

D-pinitol is a relatively new supplement that has a lot of potential for athletes and individuals following the Six-Pack Diet Plan. D-pinitol is a methyl ether of D-chiro-inositol. It is contained in pinewood and legumes, but is derived from soy for supplements. It has been shown to decrease blood sugar levels and free fatty-acid levels.

Two of D-pinitol's most significant effects for athletes are its ability to increase glucose uptake by the muscle cell and to enhance glycogen (carbohydrate storage in the muscles). This can lead to greater energy and more stable blood sugar levels. Clinical research shows that D-pinitol can increase insulin sensitivity, thereby allowing insulin to work more efficiently.

Dosage: A typical dose is 250 mg of D-pinitol taken two to three times daily with meals and one dose taken post-workout with creatine. Quality products that contain this nutrient are Meta-Cel by iSatori Global Technologies and Nitro-Tech by MuscleTech.

Fenugreek Seeds

Fenugreek seeds contain a high proportion (40 percent) of a soluble fiber known as mucilage. This fiber forms a gelatinous structure, which may slow the digestion and absorption of food from the intestine. Because of this, dietary fiber has been shown to help control blood sugar and insulin levels (and even cause weight loss to occur).

Some studies indicate a beneficial effect for fenugreek is in reducing blood glucose levels and improving glucose tolerance in patients with diabetes. In terms of weight control, the soluble fiber in fenugreek seeds can reduce dietary fat absorption by binding to fatty acids and it can create a sensation of "fullness" to reduce appetite—a good thing when trying to control blood sugar levels. There is a very interesting amino acid that is extracted from fenugreek seeds called 4-hydroxyisoleucine, which may stimulate insulin secretion and help control blood sugar.

Dosage: A typical dose is 300–500 mg of fenugreek daily, preferably after a workout and taken with carbohydrates.

Momordica Charantia (Bitter Melon Extract)

Bitter melon is an insulin-mimicking herb that can help with blood sugar regulation. It is actually derived from a common vegetable that has a bitter taste (hence the name). It lowers glucose concentration, improves glucose tolerance, and promotes glucose disposal into muscle tissue. What's interesting is that even after discontinuing this nutrient for a few weeks (after taking it for thirty days), its effects can still be seen. According to some research, it works by improving insulin secretion by the pancreas or possibly by improving the action of insulin itself. This nutrient is especially useful for people who have late-night cravings or blood sugar imbalances and has been extensively studied in diabetics.

Dosage: A typical dose is 100 mg of bitter melon (using a 4:1 standardized extract) taken one to three times daily with meals.

CONTROLLING CORTISOL LEVELS

Cortisol is necessary for many vital bodily functions, but imbalances can cause a number of effects detrimental to building a leaner body. Cortisol excess can lead to a progressive loss of protein, muscle weakness and atrophy, and a loss of bone mass. The major catabolic effects of cortisol involve facilitating the conversion of protein in muscles and connective tissue into glucose and glycogen. Cortisol can decrease the utilization of glucose by directly inhibiting glucose transport into the cells. Excess cortisol causes a redistribution of body fat to occur: basically, the extremities lose fat and muscle while the trunk and face become fatter.

Following are tips for avoiding excess cortisol levels. It's important to get your cortisol levels tested by a qualified physician before using supplements or other strategies to lower cortisol.

- Various supplemental and drug therapies may decrease cortisol levels. Helpful nutritional supplements include ginkgo biloba, vitamin A, zinc, and L-carnitine. DHEA may also help to decrease cortisol. The real challenge becomes how to control cortisol levels but not inhibit them completely because of cortisol's necessary anti-inflammatory effects. One way is to take anti-cortisol supplements in the morning upon rising and then before bedtime, as these are two times when cortisol levels seem to be higher. Timed release would not be an option because this may suppress cortisol levels over an extended period. The key is to suppress elevated levels of cortisol, not decrease normal physiological levels of this hormone, because a small amount is needed for its positive effects.

- Adjust your diet. Make sure you are supplying your body with all the essential nutrients you need for optimal function and to prevent deficiencies. This includes plenty of high-quality proteins, complex carbohydrates, essential fatty acids, vitamins, and minerals. Try not to restrict calories continuously, as some research suggests that restricting normal caloric intake by 50 percent can lead to a subsequent increase in cortisol levels. The Six-Pack Diet Plan focuses on proper nutrients in correct ratios, not calories.

- Do not overtrain. Try not to train too many days in a row without taking a day off, as this may cause cortisol levels to rise. If you are really sore, then wait an extra day, until your body fully recovers from your previous workout, before you resume training. Remember, less may be more in this case, at least in terms of cortisol. Keep workouts to under an hour and train efficiently and intensely. Listen to your body.

- Relax and try not to get stressed out easily. Take an evening walk with a loved one or take a nap when you get a chance in order to keep stress (and cortisol) levels low.

- Get seven to nine hours of sleep per night. Lack of sleep stresses the body and may cause an increase in cortisol levels. Sleep is crucial to the recovery and recuperation process and is also essential to your success on the Six-Pack Diet Plan.

- Spike insulin levels after a workout. Insulin actually interferes with cortisol and may enhance cortisol clearance from the body. Spiking insulin levels after a workout—by consuming a high-glycemic carbohydrate and protein drink—may help minimize excessive cortisol, since cortisol levels are elevated significantly after resistance training.

- Take phosphatidylserine (PS). PS is a phospholipid, a type of fat that contains the mineral phosphorus, found in every cell of the body. Research has shown that PS may be a powerful cortisol-suppressing agent. PS supplementation can blunt cortisol release significantly under stressful conditions. Taking 200–400 mg about thirty minutes before bedtime can make a huge difference in recovery. One quality PS product is Cort-Bloc from Muscle-Link.

- Supplement with vitamin C. Vitamin C is a well-known antioxidant that can also help reduce cortisol levels, according to some research. Taking 500 to 1,000 mg one hour before weight training may be helpful.

REVVING UP METABOLISM

Revving up metabolism is essential to the Six-Pack Diet Plan. The key to metabolism is the thyroid hormones. Thyroid hormones are important for normal growth and development: they maintain metabolic stability by regulating oxygen requirements, weight, and intermediary metabolism, and they affect almost all tissues of the body. Thyroid hormones also influence thermogenesis and temperature regulation, which explains some of the effects they have on energy metabolism. They may also enhance lipolysis (fat burning) in adipose tissue.

Basal metabolic rate (BMR), or the number of calories you burn at rest, is directly related to the levels of the hormones thyroxine (T4) and tri-iodothyronine (T3). Optimal thyroid activity is dependent upon a necessary level of total hormone, and the rate of conversion of T4 to T3. This conversion takes place in the liver and is regulated by the caloric intake (dietary energy) versus caloric expenditure (physical activity). In simple terms, if you are bringing in lots of fuel (food), you can turn up the heat (literally and figuratively). If you aren't bringing in enough calories, your body's thermostat is turned down, and you burn fewer calories.

Individuals who are dieting to lose "weight" can actually lower their BMR. This can be further complicated by excessive amounts of physical activity (like too much cardio). Your metabolism takes a nosedive and you are sweating away on the treadmill, yet you are at a standstill in terms of fat loss. The Six-Pack Diet Plan is designed to help you maximize metabolism and stop this from happening.

- Drink plenty of water. A recent study in *Medicine and Science in Sports and Exercise* showed that dehydration can cause a significant drop in your resting metabolic rate. Research indicates you can dehydrate up to 6 percent of your body weight during exercise. The Six-Pack Diet Plan calls for at least a gallon of water daily.

- Eat whole foods, including protein and fiber. Whole foods enhance the thermic effect of food, which can increase your metabolic rate. The thermic effect of food is the cost of metabolizing different types of food. Research indicates that a high-protein/low-fat meal boosts post-meal thermogenesis by 100 percent compared to a high-carbohydrate/low-fat meal. That's why high-protein diets are popular for weight loss.

- Eat small, frequent meals daily. Eating small meals throughout the day has been shown to be beneficial for boosting metabolism, according to clinical research. This is one of the keys to achieving fat loss success with the Six-Pack Diet Plan—eat six to eight small meals daily. Constant eating, every one-and-a-half to two hours, is one of the secrets to boosting metabolism and hence, fat loss, with the Six-Pack Diet Plan. For example, instead of a big lunch, eat half your meal and then the other half one to two hours later.

- Don't sleep too much. Getting enough sleep is important for many reasons. However, since metabolic rate can drop significantly during sleep, it is best not to exceed seven to nine hours per night.

- Train hard with weights. Research shows that weight lifting is one of the best ways to boost metabolic rate. In one study in the *Journal of Applied Physiology*, thirty men were assigned to three different exercise protocols: endurance training (jogging or running), resistance training (weights), or combined resistance and endurance training. The researchers showed that resistance training alone increases BMR and muscular strength.

THE IMPORTANCE OF SLEEP

Sleep (and what you eat before bedtime) is one of the keys to building a better body. Did you know that up to 90 percent of growth hormone secretion occurs at night? Pre-bedtime nutrition should be considered one of the essential parts of a physique-changing program. Sleep is a time for amino acid turnover and protein synthesis, as well as key hormone release. To understand this fascinating and detailed topic, it is important to understand the phenomenon of human sleep, the various hormones involved, how exercise affects these hormones, and what you can do to maximize the benefits of sleep to burn more fat.

Weight training can actually help increase fat utilization during sleep, which may lead to greater fat loss. In normal individuals, muscle growth occurs only if protein synthesis exceeds muscle protein breakdown (proteolysis). Weight training enhances the net muscle protein balance, but in the absence of proper food and supplements, it can actually create a catabolic situation (muscle breakdown). Amino acid availability is an important regulator of protein synthesis: when amino acids are present in greater amounts, muscle protein synthesis is maximized, especially when someone is weight training. One of the key times that amino acids are used to rebuild and repair muscle tissue is during sleep. So, it makes sense to give the body essential amino acids before bedtime to reduce the chances of muscle breakdown and increase protein synthesis.

Certain hormones, including growth hormone, insulin, testosterone, and cortisol, also need to be maximized to build muscle effectively and allow for optimum recovery from hard workouts. The body's circadian rhythms, which is generated by the hypothalamus (a part of the brain) in approximately 24-hour rhythms, help determine the regulation of hormone release. Resistance exercise has a profound effect on how and when these hormones are released.

Anyone involved in the Six-Pack Diet Plan should be getting seven to nine hours of sleep per night. Even partial sleep deprivation can cause alterations in the hormonal response to exercise, which can lead to major muscle breakdown—small changes in hormone output can put a halt to lean muscle building.

Stages of Sleep

What actually causes us to sleep at night? It starts with the pineal gland in the brain, which releases melatonin and this eventually converts into the hormone serotonin, causing us to fall asleep. Melatonin production is inhibited by light, so more melatonin is made at night.

Stage 1: drowsiness—often described as first in the sleep sequence; stage 1 may last for five to 10 minutes.

Stage 2: a period of light sleep— the heart rate slows and body temperature decreases; at this point, the body prepares to enter deep sleep.

Stages 3 and 4: deep sleep stages—with stage 4 being more intense than stage 3. These stages are known as slow-wave, or delta, sleep and are critical in the exercise recovery process; people who spend little time in these stages usually wake up with greater muscle soreness.

Stage 5: REM (rapid eye movement)—this is the stage of sleep when dreams occur; brain activity is actually high during this stage and the pulse increases and wave patterns in REM are similar to stage 1 sleep. Intense dreaming occurs during REM sleep as a result of heightened cerebral activity. REM sleep has several parts. The first period of REM typically lasts ten minutes, with each recurring REM stage lengthening, until the final one, typically lasting an hour.

Non-REM sleep is comprised of stages 1–4 and lasts a total of 90 to 120 minutes, with each stage clocking in at 5 to 15 minutes. Surprisingly, stages 2 and 3 repeat backwards before REM sleep is achieved. So, a normal sleep cycle has an unusual and non-cohesive pattern and occurs in the following stage sequence: 1, 2, 3, 4, 3, 2, REM. Usually, REM sleep occurs ninety minutes after sleep onset. The five stages of sleep, including their repetition, occur cyclically and a person may complete five cycles in a typical night.

Sleep, Hormones, and Muscle Building

Hormonal responses during sleep are different in weight-training individuals than sedentary individuals. For example, in resistance-trained individuals, growth hormone (GH) release is lower during the first half of sleep and higher in the second half, whereas it is the opposite in non-training individuals. Usually, testosterone is at low levels during the early part of sleep and increases as morning approaches. Cortisol is lower in the early stages of sleep but rises considerably during the second half of sleep. In exercising individuals, cortisol levels are higher during the first part of sleep and lower later on, which makes it more important to suppress cortisol in the early stages of sleep by taking key supplements before bedtime. Testosterone levels seem to rise throughout the night in training individuals. This can have huge implications for fat burning and muscle building.

It is also very important to get slow-wave sleep (stages 3 and 4), according to one study, because if you don't, it could mean a major decline in GH output—bad news for Six-Pack Dieters. The same study showed that GH secretion was associated with slow-wave sleep and that when REM sleep declined, evening cortisol levels increased.

Cell division (mitosis) in many tissues, including muscle, also shows a surge in the early hours of the morning, often coinciding with sleep stages 3 and 4. Along with the growth hormone rise, this suggests that sleep promotes general growth and repair, although it may not be sleep-dependent.

Sleep deprivation may also have a negative impact on the immune system: significant negative effects on immune function can be seen after several days of partial sleep deprivation and after only a few days of total sleep deprivation. (Free radicals may be formed when the body does not get enough sleep and can contribute to cell damage and disease.) Controlling free radicals is essential to optimal recovery from exercise, since exercise can actually increase free radicals in the body. Key antioxidants and immune-system boosters are important to take pre-bedtime.

The Bottom Line—Try and get quality sleep for maximum lean-muscle building, optimal hormone levels, increased fat loss, proper immune function, and enhanced muscle repair and recovery. This is vital to your success on the Six-Pack Diet Plan. Sleep well and you'll lose fat and gain lean body mass—lose sleep and you'll have a hard time losing fat.

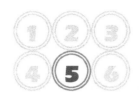

Vitamins and Minerals for Optimal Health

VITAMINS AND MINERALS ARE KEY NUTRIENTS required by the body for optimal function. Deficiencies in certain vitamins and minerals can cause serious disease states and other health problems. Unfortunately, your diet alone may not provide all the nutrients you need to stay healthy, prevent disease, and build a strong body.

The recommended dietary allowance (RDA) is a guideline designed by the United States government for the maintenance of good nutrition. The RDA is a *minimum* amount to help prevent disease, which is fine for the average person, but what about exercisers trying to get lean? This minimum amount of nutrients will not be enough for those who put their bodies through the stress of intensive training. You'll need more of these nutrients for your training and to maximize results as well as to lower the chances of illness. The Six-Pack Diet Plan will help you obtain a lean physique while also giving your body the nutrition it needs to maintain optimal health.

VITAMINS

Vitamins come in two forms: fat soluble and water soluble (the fat-soluble ones include vitamins A, D, E, and K, while the water-soluble ones are absorbed in a liquid environment and include the B vitamins). The following vitamins, taken as supplements, are essential to the Six-Pack Diet Plan.

Vitamin A

Vitamin A is also known as retinol and retinal; retinoic acid is a by-product of retinal. "Provitamin A" refers to beta-carotene, which can be converted to retinol in the body. The body uses vitamin A to support the visual cycle; cellular differentiation (which affects gene expression to control cell development); growth (appears to increase the number of receptors for growth factors); reproductive processes; bone development; and proper immune function. By boosting immune function, vitamin A may create a more favorable environment for muscle growth to occur. Vitamin A works synergistically with zinc and vitamins K and E; a deficiency of these nutrients may impair the function of vitamin A.

Food sources of vitamin A include beef liver, sweet potatoes, carrots, and spinach. Typical dosage: up to 10,000 international units (IU) in divided doses daily.

Vitamin C

Vitamin C (ascorbic acid) is an essential water-soluble vitamin and required for any intensely training athlete or dieter. It has several benefits for the body, including antioxidant properties, collagen synthesis, immuno-enhancing effects, and decreasing cortisol levels. Vitamin C helps fight free radicals, which are responsible for oxidative damage in the body. Vitamin C has been shown to considerably shorten the duration of cold episodes and the severity of symptoms. Vitamin C can help guard against illness, which is important because if you're sick, you cannot train properly and you may lose hard-earned muscle.

Vitamin C also has been shown to increase the testosterone-cortisol ratio by decreasing cortisol levels. Cortisol is a catabolic hormone that is secreted in times of stress, such as strenuous weight training. Vitamin C also aids in collagen synthesis. Collagen is a very important substance in the human body: it strengthens the skin, muscles, and bones, and is a primary component of ligaments and tendons. There are many studies that document vitamin C's importance for healthy ligaments and tendons, which can be critical for preventing injury and speeding recovery.

Vitamin C also plays a role in fat loss—it is important in the synthesis of the amino acid carnitine. Sufficient carnitine is important in fat metabolism, because carnitine helps transport long-chain fatty acids into the mitochondria where their breakdown occurs. Vitamin C also plays a key role in neurotransmitter synthesis and cholesterol catabolism.

Food sources of vitamin C include orange juice, papaya, cantaloupe, and broccoli. Typical dosage: 1–3 grams (g) in divided doses daily. There isn't a demonstrably superior form of vitamin C on the market, so ascorbic acid is fine. I would not, however, recommend the timed-release version since it may cause kidney remnants to accumulate.

Vitamin D

Vitamin D is associated with skeletal growth and strong bones. Calcitriol is considered the active form of vitamin D and functions like a steroid hormone. It plays a key role in the production of parathyroid hormone, which directs the homeostasis of blood calcium. Parathyroid hormone also stimulates calcium and phosphorus reabsorption in the kidneys. When exposed to sunlight, the body can produce it's own vitamin D.

Sources of vitamin D include sunlight and fortified milk. Typical dosage: 400 IU daily.

Vitamin E

Vitamin E includes eight different compounds synthesized by plants. Vitamin E activity is greatest in the alpha-tocopherol form (more specifically, D-alpha tocopherol). It is a fat-soluble vitamin necessary to maintain membrane integrity in body cells and acts as a powerful antioxidant, preventing the oxidation of unsaturated fatty acids in the cellular membranes. Vitamin E helps fight free radicals; there is an interrelationship between vitamin E and the mineral selenium as both are tied closely in the function of glutathione peroxidase, a powerful antioxidant. The less muscle breakdown you have by stopping damaging free radicals, the more potential muscle building that can occur. Vitamin E can be regenerated with the help of vitamin C.

A good food source of this vitamin is vegetable seed oil. Typical dosage: 400–800 IU in divided doses daily. High intakes of vitamin E can interfere with the functions of other fat-soluble vitamins, so I would not recommend taking amounts in excess of 1,200 IU daily.

Thiamine (Vitamin B_1)

Thiamine is found primarily in the form of thiamin monophosphate in the blood. Thiamine can also be converted to its phosphorylated form, thiamin diphosphate (TDP), in the body. TDP functions as a coenzyme that is necessary for generating ATP (energy). This is obviously important for promoting muscle function. Vitamin B_1 is also important in nerve conduction and appears to mimic and potentiate the effects of acetylcholine, a neurotransmitter involved in memory.

Some food sources of this vitamin include yeast, sunflower seeds, and legumes. Caffeine may inhibit the effects of thiamine. Typical dosage: 5–10 milligrams (mg) daily. Water-soluble vitamins rarely show any toxicity because excess water-soluble vitamins are excreted in the urine.

Riboflavin (Vitamin B$_2$)

Riboflavin has two coenzyme forms, flavin mononucleotide (FMN) and flavin adenine dinucleotide (FAD), which function in many metabolic reactions in the body. They can act as oxidizing agents and are a part of choline metabolism. Neurotransmitters such as dopamine require FAD for their metabolism: this can stimulate energy levels during exercise since dopamine can convert to the hormones epinephrine and norepinephrine.

Foods that have a good amount of riboflavin include beef liver, lean sirloin steak, mushrooms, and ricotta cheese. Typical dosage: 5–10 mg daily.

Niacin (Vitamin B$_3$)

Niacin, also called nicotinic acid and nicotinamide, can occur as two nucleotides, NAD and NADP. It can also be formed in the liver from the amino acid tryptophan. NAD helps produce ATP (energy), while NADP is used in a variety of processes including fatty acid synthesis, cholesterol and steroid hormone synthesis, oxidation of glutamate, and it may help reduce the oxidized form of vitamin C. Niacin has also been shown to decrease cholesterol levels. Since it acts as a vasodilator, niacin also increases vascularity (the appearance of veins). It may increase energy during a workout.

Food sources of niacin include tuna, chicken breast, and beef. Typical dosage: 50–100 mg in divided doses daily. Niacin may cause a flush (redness and vasodilation—increased blood flow), especially when taken on an empty stomach. Very high doses of niacin may also be hard on the liver. If you are concerned about these problems, you may want to try the inositol hexonicotinate form, which is easier on the liver.

Pantothenic Acid (Vitamin B$_5$)

Pantothenic acid plays an important role in energy storage as well as energy release. It is used, along with cysteine and ATP, to form coenzyme A. As a component of coenzyme A, it is essential for the production of energy from carbohydrates, fats, and protein. Some studies suggest it may also accelerate the healing process, which is important during training.

Pantothenic acid is abundant in many foods, including egg yolks and yeast. Typical dosage: 5 mg daily.

Pyridoxine (Vitamin B$_6$)

The coenzyme form of vitamin B$_6$ is associated with a vast number of enzymes as part of amino acid metabolism. Vitamin B$_6$ is also necessary to synthesize heme, the form of iron necessary for optimal blood flow and oxygenation. Niacin synthesis from tryptophan requires pyridoxal phosphate, which is one of the forms of vitamin B$_6$. It is necessary in glycogen catabolism to "unlock" carbohydrate energy, which may help reduce abdominal fat. Vitamin B$_6$ has also been shown to diminish the actions of glucocorticoid hormones (such as cortisol).

Food sources of vitamin B$_6$ include sirloin steak, navy beans, and potato. Heating, canning, freezing, or processing foods can decrease the potency of vitamin B$_6$. Typical dosage: 5–10 mg daily.

Folic Acid

Folic acid (folate) is necessary in amino acid metabolism and is also required for histidine metabolism (which prevents this amino acid from accumulating in the body; an accumulation of histidine may have adverse effects such as increased stress and anxiety). Deficiencies in this vitamin can cause muscle weakness. Ascorbic acid helps to protect folate from oxidative destruction and there is a synergistic relationship between folate and vitamin B$_{12}$ (cobalamin). This relationship is sometimes called the "methyl-folate trap" because, without vitamin B$_{12}$, folate is rendered useless in the body.

Food sources include mushrooms, spinach, and broccoli. It is easily destroyed in foods by light and heat, which may cause folate deficiencies for many people. Typical dosage: 500 micrograms (mcg) daily.

Biotin

Biotin helps many enzymes function in the body, promotes energy metabolism, and is important in the utilization of fats and amino acids.

Egg yolks contain a high amount of biotin. Egg whites contain a protein called avidin, which is unstable in heat and is deactivated; it binds to biotin and inhibits its absorption, if it is not heated. That is why it is very important to cook egg whites before eating. Typical dosage: 300–500 mcg daily.

Vitamin B$_{12}$

Vitamin B$_{12}$ (cobalamin) may boost energy levels and enhance exercise performance. Vitamin B$_{12}$ deficiency can lead to anemia.

Vitamin B$_{12}$ is usually found only in animal products; meat, fish, and poultry are good food sources of vitamin B$_{12}$. Typical dosage: 10–15 mcg daily.

Vitamin K

Vitamin K is a fat-soluble vitamin that plays an integral part in blood coagulation. It may also strengthen the bone matrix.

Food sources include leafy green vegetables and soybeans. Typical dosage: 50–100 mcg daily.

MINERALS

Minerals are the main components for enzymes and for cell function. They also help regulate the balance of fluids in the body and control the movement of nerve impulses. Recent studies show that they also can contribute to more effective fat loss.

Calcium

Calcium is the most abundant mineral in the body and about 99 percent of total body calcium is found in the bones and teeth. Calcium has various functions, such as blood clotting, nerve conduction, muscle contraction, enzyme regulation, and promoting membrane permeability. Only the ionized form of calcium is active and helps perform these functions. Calcium has also been shown to lower blood pressure. Calcium is necessary for the interaction between actin and myosin (muscle proteins), resulting in muscle contraction, so it is vital for exercisers to maintain adequate levels.

You have probably heard since you were a kid that getting enough calcium is essential to the growth and maintenance of strong bones. This is a well-known fact among the general population. However, new research has suggested that calcium has benefits to Six-Pack Dieters beyond just maintaining strong bones. Numerous studies have shown that calcium consumption may lead to significant loss of body fat. One study showed that using calcium supplements (500–2,000 mg daily) actually increased lean body mass and bone mineral density in male athletes. A 2003 study at the University of Tennessee showed that high-calcium diets can increase lipolysis (fat burning) and preserve thermogenesis during calorie restriction. They also mention that low-calcium diets can actually lead to an increase in fat.

It is not exactly known how calcium reduces body fat. One theory is that it helps block digestion and storage of body fat. Another theory is that it has positive effects on your hormones to encourage more burning of fat. Regardless, getting a full dose of 1,000 mg of calcium per day is essential for anyone striving to achieve a six-pack.

The best way to get your calcium is from skim dairy products and calcium citrate supplements. Typical dosage: 1,000–1,500 mg in divided doses daily.

Phosphorus

Phosphorus is second only to calcium in terms of its abundance in the body; approximately 85 percent of phosphorus is found in the skeleton. Most phosphorus is absorbed in the body in its inorganic phosphate form. Phosphorus is extremely important in the metabolism of energy nutrients, contributing to metabolic rate in the form of high-energy phosphate bonds such as ATP (your body's main energy source). Phosphate is also a component of the nucleic acids DNA and RNA, functions in cell membranes as phospholipids, and is involved in acid-base balance. It may act as a buffer as well, reducing lactic acid build-up. If you can delay or decrease lactic acid build-up, you may be able to train longer and not fatigue as quickly. Studies have shown that supplementing with phosphate increases endurance. Phosphate may also play a role in the formation of phosphocreatine, which can help support the production of ATP.

Meat, fish, eggs, and poultry are all good sources of phosphorus. Typical dosage: 800–1,200 mg daily.

Magnesium

Magnesium ranks fourth behind potassium in overall mineral abundance in the human body, but intracellularly it is second only to potassium. This mineral is involved in over 300 enzymatic reactions in the body, including glycolysis (the breakdown of carbohydrates into energy), the Krebs cycle, creatine phosphate formation, nucleic acid synthesis, amino acid activation, cardiac and smooth muscle contractability, cyclic AMP formation, and, most important for bodybuilders, protein synthesis. One study showed that subjects taking magnesium exhibit increases in absolute strength and lean body mass after seven weeks.

Food sources of magnesium include nuts, legumes, and soybeans. Typical dosage: 500–750 mg daily. Dietary fiber impairs magnesium absorption to a small extent, so I would recommend that you not take magnesium with any fiber source.

Sodium

Sodium is intimately involved with water balance in the body. Sodium constitutes about 93 percent of the cations (positively charged compounds that help regulate pH balance) in the blood. It helps facilitate active transport across all cellular membranes via the sodium-potassium pump. The human body generally requires around 500 mg of sodium daily. However, excess sodium intake can cause water retention in the intercellular space, giving you a bloated appearance. That is why it is important to monitor sodium intake and not take too much. The major source of sodium in the diet is generally in the form of sodium chloride (table salt).

Six-Pack Dieters need to limit high-sodium foods such as canned meats, processed foods, breads, and certain cereals. It is not advisable to completely restrict sodium intake because the hormone aldosterone may then be released and cause reabsorption of sodium in the kidneys. This will decrease sodium excretion and thus cause you to hold more water. This reabsorption generally takes about twenty-four hours, so I would recommend consuming 1,000 mg of sodium the last two weeks before trying to get really lean, and then severely restrict sodium no earlier than about eighteen hours before peaking for a contest.

Table salt, breads, cheese, and seafood are all high in sodium. Try not to exceed 2,000 mg of sodium daily.

Potassium

Potassium is a macromineral that plays an important role in the contractile functions of smooth, cardiac, and skeletal muscle. It also affects the excitability of nerve tissue and is important in maintaining electrolyte and pH balance. It is part of the sodium-potassium pump that helps transport nutrients across cellular membranes. A potassium-to-sodium ratio of 4:1 should be maintained to optimize bodily functions involving these two nutrients. Potassium can aid in decreasing or lessening muscle cramps, especially with the use of diuretics, which can cause muscle cramping.

Food sources include bananas, dates, oranges, peaches, and potatoes. Typical dosage: 2,500–4,000 mg daily.

Chloride

Chloride is the most abundant anion (negatively charged particle) in the extracellular fluid (important for pH balance). It is needed for electrolyte balance, because its negative charge neutralizes the positive charge of sodium ions with which it is usually associated. It is also required in the formation of hydrochloric acid, needed for proper digestive function.

Seafood and milk contain a good amount of chloride. Typical dosage: 1,200–1,400 mg daily.

Iron

Iron is a micromineral that is of vital importance to the human body. Iron is an essential component of hemoglobin and myoglobin, parts of the blood that transport oxygen to all the cells of the body and carbon dioxide back to the lungs where it can be expelled. A deficiency of iron may lead to anemia or a decrease in red blood cells and this can cause lower oxygenation, which may decrease exercise performance as well as lower blood flow into muscle tissue.

There are two forms of iron in food, heme and non-heme iron. Heme iron is mainly found in beef, fish, and poultry; non-heme iron is found in plant foods such as nuts, fruits, vegetables, milk, and eggs. The difference is that non-heme iron is usually bound to components of food and must be hydrolyzed prior to absorption. Heme iron is more easily absorbed than non-heme iron.

Red meats, clams, and oysters are good food sources of iron. Typical dosage: 20–30 mg daily for exercising men and 30–35 mg daily for exercising women. Ascorbic acid has been shown to enhance iron absorption and maintain iron in the appropriate state for enzyme function. Taking 1 g of ascorbic acid (vitamin C) with iron may increase absorption (especially of non-heme iron).

Zinc

Zinc is found in all organs and tissues in the human body. As a component of metalloenzymes (enzymes that contain metal ions essential to their function), it provides structural integrity to proteins. Zinc is a part of more enzyme systems than the rest of the microminerals combined. It affects many fundamental processes of life—gene expression, cell replication, membrane stabilization—and plays a structural role in hormones such as insulin, testosterone, growth hormone, and estrogen. Zinc deficiency may cause an increased susceptibility to infection and certain skin disorders.

You may have heard the old folktale that eating oysters will put you in a "loving mood" (that is, enhance your libido), and actually there is science behind this claim. Oysters are an excellent source of highly absorbable zinc, and several studies have found that zinc consumption is essential for boosting testosterone. One study showed that six months of zinc supplementation actually doubled testosterone levels.

If boosting testosterone isn't reason enough to make sure you are getting enough zinc, this mineral has numerous other benefits for Six-Pack Dieters. Many studies have shown that zinc supplementation may be a potent immune booster that can reduce the severity and symptoms of colds. Since intense exercise can increase your chances of catching a cold (enhanced stress from exercise compromises proper immune function), this immune-enhancing effect is highly important to those who exercise on a regular basis.

Oysters, beef liver, and wheat germ are all good food sources of zinc. Typical dosage: 25–30 mg daily.

Copper

Copper is an enzyme activator in crucial reactions such as the anti-inflammatory process and the synthesis of connective tissue. Copper status strongly affects the levels of neuropeptides, enkephalins, and endorphins, which help boost immune function and the response to stress.

Good food sources of copper include liver, shellfish, and whole grains. Typical dosage: 2–4 mg daily. There is an antagonistic relationship between copper and zinc, which is why I would not recommend taking copper with zinc but rather separately, at different times of the day, and with food.

Selenium

Selenium is an essential cofactor of glutathione peroxidase, a powerful antioxidant enzyme. It is also involved in pancreatic and immune system function, DNA repair and enzyme activation, and detoxification of heavy metals. Selenium is also necessary for iodine metabolism, which acts in the conversion of T4 to triiodothyronine (T3), the active form of thyroid hormone. Selenium may also act as an insulin mimicker, which can help with blood sugar regulation and possibly inhibit fat storage. (Selenomethionine is the best form for supplementation as it has been researched more thoroughly on cancer and immune system support.)

Some food sources of selenium include grains, meat, and poultry. Typical dosage: 150–200 mcg daily.

Chromium

Chromium acts to form glucose tolerance factor, which helps insulin bind to its receptor. This action will affect cellular glucose uptake and intracellular carbohydrate and lipid metabolism, which can help improve nutrient uptake into muscle tissue, thus lowering fat storage. Chromium may play a role in lipid and cholesterol metabolism by affecting lipoprotein lipase activity. Some studies show it improves blood lipid profiles and causes fat loss.

Food sources of chromium include cinnamon, brewer's yeast, and mushrooms. Typical dosage: 400–800 mcg in divided doses daily.

Iodide

Iodide's main function is in the synthesis of the thyroid hormones by the thyroid gland. Thyroid hormones stimulate metabolism, oxygen consumption, and heat production. Iodide thus possibly supports fat loss by increasing metabolism.

Seafood, sunflower seeds, and mushrooms are all good food sources of iodide. Typical dosage: 150 mcg daily.

Manganese

Manganese functions both as an enzyme activator and as a constituent of metalloenzymes. A deficiency can cause impaired growth. It increases superoxide dismutase activity (SOD), a powerful antioxidant that may help with the healing process.

Food sources include wheat bran, legumes, and nuts. Typical dosage: 15–20 mg daily.

Molybdenum

Molybdenum is a cofactor for four metalloenzymes (xanthine dehydrogenase, aldehyde oxidase, xanthine oxidase, and sulfide oxidase) that function in many different reactions in the human body.

Soybeans and pasta are some food sources of molybdenum. Typical dosage: 150–200 mcg daily.

Fluorine

The major effects of fluorine or fluoride (which is fluorine bound to either a metal, non-metal, or organic compound) are related to the mineralization of bones and teeth. (Mineralization is the process of forming a mineral by combination of a metal with another element; also, the process of converting a bone into a mineral.) It may decrease bone resorption (loss of minerals from the bone), so it is often used to treat osteoporosis.

Some food sources include mackerel and sardines. Typical dosage: 2–4 mg daily.

Silicon

Silicon plays a vital role in the formation of bones, connective tissue, and cartilage. It hastens mineralization of bones as well as promotes growth. Silicon has a positive influence on collagen synthesis and is also needed to form glycosaminoglycans, components of the fluid around joints.

Food sources include many plant foods, including beets and turnips. Typical dosage: 15–20 mg daily.

Vanadium

Vanadium is both water- and fat-soluble and is present in all healthy tissue. Vanadium may have some insulin-mimicking properties: it can stimulate glucose uptake into cells and enhances glucose metabolism for glycogen synthesis, which can support energy levels and help transport key nutrients into muscle tissue.

Foods contain very little vanadium, so supplementation may be necessary. Typical dosage: 10 mg daily. The vanadate form is up to five times more efficiently absorbed than vanadyl.

Boron

Boron influences the composition, structure, and strength of bones and also plays a role in how certain minerals (such as calcium) are metabolized.

Fruits and vegetables, such as apples, raisins, and lettuce, contain boron. Typical dosage: 2–3 mg daily.

TIPS FOR MAXIMIZING VITAMIN AND MINERAL USAGE

- A good multivitamin/multimineral product can provide efficacious amounts of the nutrients described above. At the very least, make sure you're providing your body with the minimum recommended dietary allowance (RDA) for each nutrient. Some good supplements include Opti-Pack by Super Nutrition and Mega Men by GNC.

    Tips to remember when taking supplements on the Six-Pack Diet Plan:

- Take the fat-soluble vitamins A, D, E, and K with essential fatty acids (such as olive oil or flaxseed oil) to allow for better absorption, since these vitamins work with fats and in cell membranes, which protect the cell.

- Take vitamins E and C together as they seem to have a synergistic antioxidant effect.

- The body can only absorb and effectively retain about 250 mg of vitamin C at one time, so it's best to take divided doses.

- Vitamin C should be taken about one hour prior to exercise and right after exercise as well.

- Use the natural form of vitamin E, D-alpha tocopherol, as it is better absorbed and retained by the body, instead of the synthetic form, DL-alpha tocopherol.

- Do not take chitosan or other "fat blockers" with the fat-soluble vitamins (A, D, E, and K), as absorption of these vitamins can be negatively affected with these products.

- Beta-carotene can take the place of vitamin A. It is better to use beta-carotene to achieve a higher level of carotenoids, especially if you're concerned about excessive intakes of vitamin A. Pregnant women, for example, should not consume vitamin A.

- The B vitamins, such as vitamin B_6 and vitamin B_{12}, should be taken before exercise to enhance energy levels.

- Niacin (vitamin B_3) can cause a skin flush or irritation, but using the niacinamide form eliminates this effect. "Slow release" niacin has the potential for greater toxicity and adverse effects to the liver, so avoid it.

- People taking prescription warfarin (Coumadin), an anti-coagulant agent, should not take high levels of vitamin K.

- Women taking oral contraceptives need extra folic acid.

- Calcium should be taken with vitamin D to increase absorption rate and retention. Take calcium separately from magnesium; calcium and magnesium compete for absorption.

- Consult your health-care practitioner regarding your iron intake. There are no real requirements or deficiencies of iron in men; however, due to menstruation, women should discuss supplementation with their doctors if they are prone to iron anemia deficiency. This can often be resolved with a supplementary intake of iron.

- Take more zinc for a "T-boost": zinc plays a key role in testosterone levels, so *men* should try and consume at least 30 mg daily. (Copper competes with zinc for absorption, so it is best not to take zinc and copper together.)

- Don't underestimate the importance of selenium. Selenium is very important in helping to regulate metabolism as it supports the conversion of inactive thyroid (T4) to active thyroid (T3) hormone.

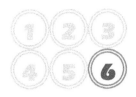

The Six-Pack Training Program

ESS IS MORE—THAT IS THE KEY to the Six-Pack Training Program with regard to both cardiovascular exercise and weight training. The Six-Pack philosophy for maximum fat loss and lean muscle gains is short, intense workouts using maximal weights. Research shows that intense weight-lifting sessions build more muscle, more quickly.

The cardio work on the Six-Pack Training Program also emphasizes intensity. Sprints, performed in the morning on an empty stomach, are the key to boosting fat loss. Traditional cardio of longer duration is then done once per week.

The Six-Pack Training Program will help you get the results you want, fast. And because of the emphasis on intensity of workouts rather than duration, the Six-Pack Training Program fits easily into your busy schedule.

SIX-PACK CARDIOVASCULAR WORKOUT

For cardiovascular work, the Six-Pack Training Program calls for something more radical than the traditional moderately paced walk in the park. On the Six-Pack Training Program, you'll sprint two times a week, first thing in the morning on an empty stomach (drinking plenty of water first, of course). Research clearly shows that fat burning is suppressed significantly when carbohydrates are ingested more than six hours before exercise. Because of this, cardiovascular work on an empty stomach can help burn up to three times more fat.

When insulin is elevated, such as after eating, it can inhibit the fat-loss process. In a fasting state, insulin levels are low. So, by performing cardio on an empty stomach, your body is in prime fat-burning mode. Also, wait an hour after the cardio workout to eat, as this will allow for further metabolism increases and fat loss. Make sure you drink plenty of water before, during, and after cardio.

Research shows that high-intensity exercise like sprinting can burn more fat than low-intensity cardio work and help maintain lean muscle mass as well. Have you noticed how Olympic sprinters, though lean, are very muscular, while long-distance runners are simply skinny? Well, those sprinters are definitely onto something.

However, since moderate-paced cardio for a longer period of time does have many benefits, one day a week you will perform cardio first thing in the morning for thirty-five to forty minutes at a moderate pace (like a brisk walk or a jog). Again, waiting an hour after the cardio workout to eat can allow greater fat burning to occur.

For the sprints, you only have to run for twelve minutes per session, but intensity is the key. Alternate a thirty-second, all-out sprint with a ninety-second walk, until you reach twelve minutes total workout time. Obviously, you'll probably have to work up to this level. You can start with six minutes total and then increase the time. So, perform three days of cardio per week—two days of sprinting first thing in the morning on an empty stomach and one day of moderate-paced cardio—for the best results in lowering body fat. Always be sure to stretch and warm up before and after the cardio workout.

WHY WEIGHT TRAINING IS IMPORTANT

Some dieters ask, "Why should I lift weights?" and then insist on doing cardio only; however, it is very important to weight train to lose fat and maintain lean body mass. In fact, intense training with weights is vital. A thorough review of the research on weight training shows that intensity builds muscle and causes fat loss. That's right, what "hardcore" trainers instinctively knew has been confirmed by many research studies, and it makes sense physiologically and practically. Shorter, more intense workouts rev up the body's metabolic engine better than longer workouts with lots of rest between sets. They also increase anabolic hormones, which are the key to lean muscle mass gain and fat loss.

Here's a review of some of the applicable studies on weight training:

• One study entitled "Blood hormone and metabolite levels during graded cycle ergometer exercise" published back in 1985 showed that there was an increase in adrenaline, noradrenaline, growth hormone (GH), cyclic AMP (cAMP or cyclic adenosine monophosphate), and lactate after increasing exercise workload. In other words, as the amount of resistance (weight) increased, the greater was the anabolic hormone response. When you increase lactic acid output (that burning sensation you get in the muscles after reaching training fatigue), you correspondingly increase cAMP. This causes an increase in growth hormone levels, which can lead to greater lean body mass and fat loss. Cyclic AMP is formed from ATP (adenosine triphosphate) and an accumulation of lactic acid can boost cAMP formation. Cyclic AMP helps hormones trigger target cells, activates enzymes, and is a key factor in hormone modification, muscle building, and fat loss.

- Another study comparing low- and high-intensity trainers, published in the *Journal of Clinical Endocrinology and Metabolism,* showed that after only ten minutes of high-intensity exercise, GH levels were elevated in the men who performed high-intensity training. Those in the high-intensity group were causing muscle fatigue to occur, which led to a corresponding increase in GH levels, significantly above the levels seen in the low-intensity exercisers.

- A study in the *Journal of Applied Physiology* confirmed the results of the previous study. It showed that shorter rest periods between sets (one minute vs. three minutes) caused a rise in GH levels. Again, lactic acid levels were elevated in these subjects. The study concluded that more intense exercise may increase GH levels.

- A study conducted at Pennsylvania State University concluded that "higher volumes of total work [specifically high-intensity workouts] produce significantly greater increases in circulating anabolic hormones during the recovery phase following exercise." It showed increases in both testosterone and GH levels secondary to higher volume (resistance) weight training. Testosterone, a steroid hormone that regulates male reproductive function, is called the most powerful muscle-building hormone because it increases muscle protein synthesis and net muscle protein balance, resulting in increased muscle mass.

- A University of Kansas study published in the *Journal of Applied Physiology* in 1998 compared the effects of resistance training, aerobic training, or both resistance and aerobic training, on BMR (basal metabolic rate). The results showed something fairly remarkable that went against conventional beliefs: resistance training alone (just three days a week of intense training with short rest periods between sets) will increase BMR and muscular strength. It showed that resistance training can boost metabolism (and hence fat loss) much more effectively than endurance training alone.

- A more recent Japanese study published in June 2003 in the *Journal of Sports Medicine and Physical Fitness* looked at the effects of "supersets" on GH secretion in men—comparing intense weight-training regimens with or without a burnout set afterward. The men who performed a quick burnout set after a heavy set of resistance exercise consistently had a greater increase in GH secretion versus men who didn't do an additional burnout set. So, lactic acid release from the extra burnout set is bene - ficial in boosting GH levels. Keep in mind that GH also has some very powerful anti-aging benefits.

- Another study published in June 2003 in the journal *Medicine and Science in Sports and Exercise* showed that concentric (quick, explosive, muscle-shortening) weight training boosts GH and can also increase testosterone levels. The shorter rest times between sets were important to boosting lactate and GH levels. The concentric movements in this study were compared to eccentric (muscle-lengthening) movements and shown to be better for increasing GH levels.

As you can see, many studies confirm the benefits of short, intense training sessions like those recommended in the Six-Pack Training Program. This also makes training very convenient and time efficient.

SIX-PACK GUIDELINES FOR RESISTANCE TRAINING

1. Train one body part per workout. The one exception is the arms—you can train biceps and triceps together. Concentrate on contracting each working muscle.

2. Perform about three exercises per body part, with one set to maximum failure (and sometimes beyond) in each exercise.

3. Use explosive movements and focus on the eccentric phase (lowering

or muscle-lengthening part of the movement) with fairly maximal weights.

4. Workouts should last around forty-five minutes at the most. Use your full mental focus and concentration during lifts.

5. Take plenty of rest days. Many natural trainers tend to overtrain, which can in many cases be worse than under-training. Train smarter, not harder.

6. Perform lots of strenuous stretching before, during, and after the workout. It may actually be uncomfortable sometimes to stretch this hard, but it really makes a difference in lean muscle mass.

FIVE WEIGHT-TRAINING TIPS

1. **Use Free weights**—Examples include barbells and dumbbells. These free movements work large muscle groups and also engage stabilizer muscles creating a more balanced body.

2. **Use Machines**—Examples include cables and pre-set machines in the gym. These help isolate smaller muscle groups like the biceps. They can help increase definition and muscle detail.

3. **Breathing**—It is very important to breathe properly while training and NEVER hold your breath during an exercise movement. The general rule is to breathe out all your air on the contraction phase (concentric) of a movement while breathing in on the lowering phase of an exercise (eccentric). So for example on bench press, you would breathe all your air out while pressing the weight up and breathe in while bringing the weight down.

4. **Use a Spotter**—A spotter is someone who watches you and can help you while you perform a movement. This is vitally important for safety reasons but a good spotter can also help push you to your limit while training. There is definitely power in numbers when it comes to weight training. Training with a few people can certainly add motivation.

5. **Warm-Up**—By doing some light aerobic activity about 5-10 minutes before weight training, you can help lower the chances for injury and allow your muscles to be better prepared for resistance exercise.

Weight Training and Women

There is a common myth that hard weight training will cause women to bulk up. This is simply not true, according to extensive research. Women have about one-tenth the level of testosterone of men and, depending on their diet, will not bulk up by lifting weights. Women and men should train similarly in the weight room. The Six-Pack Diet Plan can help both men and women achieve a lean, healthy physique.

SIX-PACK TRAINING SCHEDULE

What follows is the Six-Pack weight training routine. The timing of the actual workout can vary, but I suggest cardio in the morning and weight training in the late afternoon. Some people prefer the morning for weights, as it matches up better with the individual's natural circadian rhythms (i.e., higher energy and testosterone levels). Always consult a physician before starting any training program.

The routine is basically a ten-day weight training/cardio cycle. The premise of the plan is to train one body part per workout daily, except for biceps and triceps, which you will train together. Cardio is performed three times during that ten-day cycle. There are also two days off for rest during this ten-day intense training phase. Begin each workout with a ten-minute warm-up, such as walking on the treadmill.

Be sure to follow the exact routine outlined below. Beginners, or those who haven't trained in a while, should use lighter weights and do moderate cardio (a brisk walk for thirty minutes) during the first two ten-day cycles.

DAY ONE

Cardio in the morning: sprinting (intense sprints alternating with walking)

Chest

Incline barbell press. Using an incline barbell bench, grasp the bar with a shoulder-width grip and bring the bar down to the top part of the chest (about two inches from actually touching your chest). Then, press the bar all the way to the top again while keeping your elbows back and your back arched/chest up.

One set of fifteen repetitions (reps)

One set of eight reps

One set to absolute failure

Note: The tempo on the last set should always be 2:0:X. That is, 2 seconds on the eccentric, or muscle-lengthening phase of the movement, no pause, and X, with X meaning as fast as you can lift the weight on the concentric, or quick, explosive muscle-shortening part of the movement. The amount of rest between sets should be about sixty to ninety seconds. For the absolute failure set, use as heavy a weight as possible for at least six to eight repetitions.

Dumbbell bench press. Grab two dumbbells and lie down on a flat bench. Bring the weight down close to your body and keep your elbows back. Press the weight back up, keeping your back arched and chest up; contract your arms and chest at the top of the movement.

One set of fifteen reps

One set of eight reps

One set to absolute failure

Dumbbell fly. Lie down on a flat bench with two dumbbells. Bring the weight down, using a wide range of motion. Bring the weight back up as if you are giving a large person a big bear hug and slightly point your pinky fingers inward. Make sure your back is arched and your chest is up. If you "cave in" your chest, then you will mainly be using your shoulders.

One set of fifteen reps

One set to absolute failure

Dips. Using a dip bar at a gym, keep your elbows by your sides and lean forward to a forty-five-degree angle, pushing your body up and down, contracting the chest. If you are not at a gym, sit on the edge of a couch or bed. Straighten your legs and go forward while keeping your hands on the couch or bed. Bend at the elbows and raise your body up and down.

One set to absolute failure with added weight, if needed. Assisted dips on a machine can also be performed.

DAY TWO

Back

Wide-grip pull-up to the front. Using a pull-up bar, get a grip that is slightly wider than your shoulders and pull your body up to where you can almost touch your chest to the bar. Go all the way down and repeat.

Three sets of ten reps (work up to that level if you can't do that many at first)

Barbell bent-over row (shoulder-width grip). Using a barbell, get an over-hand shoulder-width grip. Bend forward at the waist, keep your head up, and extend the bar as low as you can. Then pull it back up to the lower part of your waist/abdominal region while keeping your back straight and your knees slightly bent.

One set of twelve reps

One set of eight reps

One set to absolute failure

Seated cable row. Using the seated cable row machine and a V-grip bar, pull the bar toward the lower part of your abs while keeping your elbows by your side. Extend to the point where your arms are straightened and repeat. Keep your back straight and stationary throughout the movement.

One set of fifteen reps

One set to absolute failure

DAY THREE

Cardio, at a moderate pace (thirty-five to forty minutes): walking or jogging

Abs

Lying crunch. On a mat, lie on your back with your knees bent. Place your hands behind your head but do not lock your fingers together. Crunch up, breathing out, as high as you can go without lifting your lower back off the ground. In fact, try to 'press' your lower back into the ground on the crunch. Feel the abs contracting and repeat.

Two sets of twenty reps

Hanging leg raise. Hang by your arms on a pull-up bar or use a machine. Raise your legs up with your knees slightly bent until your thighs are about parallel to the ground, then lower your legs. Repeat.

Three sets of twenty-five reps

Lying side crunch. Lie on your side and place your hands behind your head (do not lock) and roll your body upward, squeezing the oblique muscles (the muscles next to your abs on the sides). Repeat on other side.

Three sets of fifteen reps each side

Machine crunch with weight. Using a crunch machine, lean forward with the weight pad placed against your chest and squeeze the abdominal muscles, breathing out on the way down.

One set of ten reps

Day Four

Shoulders

Barbell shoulder press to the front. Using a straight bar and a shoulder-width overhand grip, press the bar overhead and bring down to the front at about chin level and press up again. Keep your lower back pressed against the bench seat with your back arched.

One set of fifteen to twenty reps

One set of eight reps

One set to absolute failure

Barbell shrug. Using a straight bar, get an overhand grip about shoulder width apart. Shrug the shoulders up, trying to touch your ears, focusing on the trapezius (upper back) muscle, then repeat. Do not roll your shoulders back—it should be a straight up and down motion. Use maximum weight as you are only going up a few inches. It can be beneficial in this movement to use wrist straps to secure the bar and enhance grip.

One set of fifteen reps

One set of eight reps

One set to absolute failure

Dumbbell side lateral. Using two dumbbells, start by keeping them together (palms facing each other) in front of you. Lift the two dumbbells out to the side until your arms are parallel to the ground, with your arms slightly bent, then repeat. This exercise focuses on the side deltoid muscles (the side part of your shoulders).

One set of fifteen reps

One set of eight reps

One set to absolute failure

Dumbbell rear lateral. While sitting on the end of a bench, lean forward and bend down. Hold two dumbbells together (palms facing each other) and lift up behind you with arms slightly bent. Use a wide arc motion.

One set of fifteen reps

One set to absolute failure

DAY FIVE

Cardio in the morning: sprinting

Biceps and Triceps

Standing barbell curl. Using a straight barbell, take an underhand shoulder-width grip and curl the bar upward while keeping the elbows right by your side. Contract the biceps at the top and repeat. Try not to swing the weight up, although on the heavier weight it is okay to slightly cheat (but only for experienced lifters).

One set of fifteen to twenty reps

One set of eight reps

One set to absolute failure

Preacher curl. Sitting on a preacher bench, grab an E-Z curl bar using an underhand grip with your hands close together. With your elbows against the pad, curl the weight up, contract the biceps at the top of the movement then repeat.

One set of fifteen reps

One set to absolute failure

Incline dumbbell curl. Using a forty-five-degree incline bench, lie down on your back with two dumbbells of equal weight in your hands (palms facing each other at the bottom of the curl movement). With your head resting against the pad, curl the weights up together in one swift motion, turning the dumbbell slightly outward at the top to really squeeze the bicep at the peak. Keep your elbows in and close to your sides throughout the movement. Repeat.

One set to absolute failure

Lying tricep press with E-Z curl bar. On a flat bench, lie down on your back and have a workout partner hand you the E-Z curl bar. Grab the bar using an overhand close grip (with hands close together). Bring the bar to the top of your head while keeping your elbows in, then press upward to the top in an arc motion. Repeat and make sure to breathe throughout the movement. If you have minor elbow problems, using a decline bench instead of a flat one can help.

One set of fifteen to twenty reps

One set of eight reps

One set to absolute failure

Tricep pushdown using the straight bar. On the cable machine, use a straight bar. Grab the bar with a close overhand grip. Stand close to the bar and push the bar down until you can lock and fully contract your triceps. Keep your elbows by your side and bring the weight up to the point where your forearms are parallel to the ground, then press down again.

One set of fifteen reps

One set to absolute failure

Tricep pushdown with rope. Use the same motion as with the straight bar, but use the rope attachment to the cable machine and hold the rope at the bottom.

One set to absolute failure

DAY SIX

Day off

DAY SEVEN

 ## Legs

Free barbell squat. Use a straight barbell and place it on the lower part of your trapezius muscle (right above where the trapezius meets the rhomboids—that is, the upper part of the back below the bottom of the neck). Take a shoulder-width stance with your toes pointed out slightly (to take some stress off your knees). While keeping your back straight, chest up, and head looking straight ahead, squat down to where your quadriceps (thighs) are about parallel to the ground, then come back up while squeezing the leg muscles. Try not to lean forward and remember to breathe throughout the movement. This exercise should be performed on a safety/power rack with a competent spotter.

One set of fifteen to twenty reps

One set of eight reps

One set to absolute failure

Note: The Smith machine can be used for squats if balance is a problem. (The Smith machine is a machine that can perform compound movements yet provides added safety.)

Leg press. Use the leg press machine, placing your feet (toes pointing outward slightly) on the machine about shoulder-width apart. Take the weight off of the safety pads using the lever(s) and bring the weight down as low as possible, then press back up. It is very important to breathe throughout and have a competent spotter.

One set of fifteen reps
or

Barbell lunge. Using a straight barbell (or the Smith machine), get under the bar as if you were going to do squats. Place one leg forward with a wide stance (like taking a giant step forward). Keep the foot there and bend at the knee to where it is at about a ninety-degree angle, then return to the starting position and repeat. Take a break between legs and then repeat with the other leg forward.

One set of eight reps

One set to absolute failure

Leg extension. Use the leg extension machine, keeping your feet evenly positioned. Contract the quadriceps at the top of the movement and use a full range of motion.

One set to absolute failure (about ten to fifteen reps)

Stiff-legged deadlift. Using a barbell, take an overhand shoulder-width grip. With your feet close together and toes pointed slightly outward, bend down with your knees slightly bent, bring the bar to your ankles, and then come back up again. Make sure to keep your back straight and *do not* round your back. Keep the bar close to your legs as you perform the exercise, and breathe!

One set of fifteen reps

One set of eight reps

One set to absolute failure

Lying leg curl. Using the lying leg curl machine, lie down flat on your stomach and curl the weight up using the back of the legs while pointing the toes away from you. Make sure to use a full range of motion when bending the leg.

One set to absolute failure

Standing calf raise. Using the standing calf raise machine, keep your toes pointing straight ahead and your feet about six inches apart on the bottom platform. Place your shoulders under the weighted pad, and lift up and down using the calf muscles. Keep your knees locked as much as possible or at most only slightly bent. Make sure to extend all the way down and then all the way up.

One set of fifteen to twenty reps

One set of twelve to fifteen reps

One set to absolute failure

DAY EIGHT

Chest routine (refer to Day One)

DAY NINE

Cardio in the morning: sprinting
Abs routine (refer to Day Three)

DAY TEN

Day off.

Repeat Cycle

Incorporating these short, intense workouts of the Six-Pack Training Program into your daily routine can help you achieve the lean and strong body you desire.

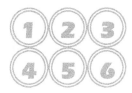

Putting It All Together

NOW THAT YOU HAVE EXTENSIVE INFORMATION on the scientific basis of the Six-Pack Diet Plan, it is time to put together all the pieces of the puzzle and get a complete plan to maximize fat loss permanently. Please remember that the Six-Pack Diet Plan is not a short-term fad diet but rather a results-oriented fat-loss solution. It requires commitment and long-term adherence for absolute success. The plan has three phases—an initial "get lean" phase, an optional, one-week peak-physique phase, and a maintenance phase.

PHASE 1: GETTING LEAN

Phase 1 lasts eleven weeks and requires mental focus, commitment, and consistency to achieve fat-loss success.

STEP 1

Figure out caloric intake and daily nutrients. To do this, multiply your current body weight by ten calories to determine how many calories you need to consume daily. The recommended Six-Pack macronutrient ratio is 45 percent protein, 40 percent carbohydrates, and 15 percent essential fats. For example, if you are a 200-pound male, you will need to consume around 2,000 calories daily, separated into many small meals throughout the day. Here's how it breaks down:

Total Calories:

200 (pounds) $\times$ 10 (calories) = consume 2,000 calories daily

Protein:

45 percent protein = 2,000 $\times$ 0.45 = 900 total calories from protein daily

900 calories of protein/4 calories per gram of protein = 225 grams (g) protein daily

Carbohydrates:

40 percent carbohydrates = 2,000 $\times$ 0.40 = 800 total calories from carbohydrates

800 calories of carbohydrates $\div$ 4 calories per gram of carbohydrates = 200 g carbs daily

TIP: Remember to consume a good portion of these carbs first thing in the morning and after a hard workout.

Fat:

15 percent fat = 2,000 $\times$ 0.15 = 300 total calories from fat daily

300 calories of fat/9 calories per gram of fat = 33 g fat daily

DAILY CALORIE BREAKDOWN—LEAN PHASE				
Bodyweight (lbs)	Total Daily Calories	Protein (grams)	Carbohydrates (grams)	Fat (grams)
100	1,000	112.5	100	17
120	1,200	135.0	120	20
140	1,400	157.5	140	23
160	1,600	180.0	160	27
180	1,800	202.5	180	30
200	2,000	225.0	200	33
220	2,200	247.5	220	37
240	2,400	270.0	240	40
260	2,600	292.5	260	43
280	2,800	315.0	280	47
300	3,000	337.5	300	50

STEP 2

Divide up your daily meals so that a majority of your carbohydrates are consumed in the first meal and the meal right after training. Eat six to eight small meals daily. This helps increase the thermogenic effect of foods and modulates insulin levels to discourage fat storage. Use meal-replacement powders and protein bars for convenience. (See Chapter 2.)

STEP 3

Use supplements to increase thermogenesis, modify hormones, and achieve lean abs with the diet and training program. (See Chapters 3 and 4.)

STEP 4

Eat only protein and fiber during the four hours before bedtime. Since metabolism is generally slower at this time, keeping insulin levels low by not eating too many carbohydrates can help you reduce fat storage and maximize growth hormone release during sleep.

STEP 5

Watch your sodium intake. When you retain water you hide your abdominal definition. High-sodium foods include gravies, sauces, soups, breads, canned meats, and condiments like ketchup.

STEP 6

Drink at least one gallon of water daily. Tip: Fill a gallon jug of water every morning and make sure it is finished by day's end.

STEP 7

Eat slowly and make sure to chew your food well. This will allow your food to be better digested and utilized by the body.

STEP 8

Take a multivitamin/mineral and/or other nutrients for optimal body function during the Six-Pack Diet Plan. (See Chapter 5.)

STEP 9

Start cardiovascular and resistance training using short, intense workouts, as outlined in Chapter 6.

PHASE 2: PEAK PHYSIQUE (OPTIONAL)

One of the questions I constantly get asked is, "How do I get real lean for a contest or photo shoot?" With the Six-Pack Diet Plan, this one-week phase is specifically designed to get you super lean and into the best shape of your life. It is an *optional phase* and is intended only for those people looking to peak in terms of leanness—that is, in preparation for a photo shoot or contest. If you are not interested in "peaking" but simply want to continue with the Six-Pack Diet Plan, then skip this phase and move to the maintenance phase (phase 3) outlined below.

By this time, you've worked hard for eleven weeks on the Six-Pack Diet Plan. You gave up sleep at least three times a week to do your morning cardio work. You religiously took all your supplements throughout the program. You can now see the light at the end of the tunnel. But you can improve your physique by 10 to 20 percent by following phase 2 of the Six-Pack Diet Plan.

There are some simple and detailed guidelines that, if followed properly, can lead to a peak physique. I have peaked for photos and natural bodybuilding competitions for the past ten years and have helped dozens of other people do it, too. What you are about to read are my "secrets" to physique peaking based on this experience and sound scientific research.

Please note that recommended dosages for foods and supplements are general recommendations and should be adjusted for weight. If you have any medical conditions, consult a physician before trying any of these "peaking" tips. These techniques require work and commitment, but since you have committed to the Six-Pack Diet Plan, why not do everything right, especially at the end? Anything worth achieving takes hard work and effort.

During the last week, there are three main goals for physique peaking:

• Maintain as much lean muscle mass as possible.

• Lose that last bit of body fat.

- Get rid of excess body water to allow your muscles to appear super ripped (the "dry" look as it's referred to in bodybuilding circles).

Let's investigate how these three goals can be maximized in one week.

MAINTAINING LEAN MUSCLE MASS

Maintaining lean muscle mass requires consuming plenty of high-quality protein. The protein sources I recommend are orange roughy fish, low-sodium tuna, egg whites, and chicken breast. These are good sources of protein that are low in fat and have relatively low sodium (sodium causes water retention and thus should be reduced during phase 2). Proteins supply amino acids needed for building lean muscle.

It is also important to consume anti-catabolic supplements that can help maintain lean muscle and lower muscle breakdown, especially in a calorie-restrictive diet plan. These include phosphatidylserine and BCAAs (branched chain amino acids). You can take these products as late as up until the night before a contest.

Phosphatidylserine (PS)—Cortisol levels (a catabolic hormone) can soar during hard training and dieting. PS has been shown to help suppress cortisol levels so muscle breakdown can be minimized. Dosage: 400 milligrams (mg) after weight training and/or 400 mg before bedtime.

Branched-chain amino acids (BCAAs)—These special amino acids (leucine, isoleucine, and valine) act directly in potentiating protein synthesis, minimizing muscle breakdown, sparing protein, and even reducing abdominal fat, according to a study published in the *International Journal of Sports Medicine*. Dosage: 5 g daily, taken in two divided doses (preferably after a workout and before bedtime).

LOSING BODY FAT

You can't lose a lot of body fat during the last week before a contest, but you can lose some of that last bit that may be left. Here are tips for doing that:

- Continue using thermogenic fat-loss supplements. One tip is to add pure cayenne pepper to each meal. (You can find it in the spice section of your local grocery store.) Cayenne pepper can increase metabolism and body temperature and may help aid in fat loss.

- Your meals should be very low in fat and should consist of low-fat, low-sodium proteins, a complex carbohydrate source, and fibrous vegetables, such as broccoli and cauliflower.

- Do a cardio workout at least twice this week.

GETTING RID OF EXCESS WATER

It is very important to consume one to one and a half gallons of water daily to help flush out toxins and excess sodium, allowing muscles to appear

Seven Tips to Reduce Abdominal Fat

Tip #1—Do cardio: By performing cardiovascular work three to four times a week, you can burn more calories and increase metabolic rate. This can help lower body fat and allow you to see more definition in your abdominal region.

Tip #2—Train with weights: We all know that exercise helps burn calories, but your metabolism is also increased for up to nine hours after just one weight-training session. Perform exercises like crunches and leg raises (hanging from a bar or lying on a bench): by targeting the upper and lower abdominal muscles, you will be on your way to a six-pack.

Tip #3—Take conjugated linoleic acid (CLA): CLA seems to work as a repartitioning agent; that is, it reduces body fat without changing body weight. Research shows that CLA can significantly reduce abdominal fat. It seems to work specifical-

ly on brown adipose tissue located deep in the abdomen. A typical dose is anywhere between 1.4 and 4 g daily.

Tip #4—Lower cortisol levels: A major risk factor for increasing abdominal fat is the hormone cortisol. Cortisol causes a redistribution of body fat and specifically increases belly fat. Abdominal fat (both white and brown fat) has up to four times more cortisol receptors than fat in other parts of the body. Due to these receptors, abdominal fat is very sensitive to the fat-increasing effects of circulating cortisol. Belly fat tissue actually increases in size when it is exposed to cortisol. Reducing stress and getting enough sleep every night can certainly help in managing cortisol levels. In a study published in the *Tufts University Health & Nutrition Letter,* individuals who slept seven hours or less tighter. Increased cell volume created by extra water intake is a good thing as well. Try drinking distilled water for five days before the contest or photo shoot to lower daily sodium intake. About sixteen hours beforehand, lower your water intake drastically and only sip water as needed (to facilitate the taking of supplements or to "wet the whistle"). You should only drink about 16 ounces of water during the last twelve to sixteen hours before an event to insure that excess body water can be eliminated.

To further help flush out the system, it is beneficial to take a natural herbal diuretic, such as dandelion root, starting about three days before

---

per night had greater levels of cortisol in the afternoon than when they slept nine hours a night. Try to get nine hours of sleep every night. There are also some powerful supplements that can stop cortisol in its tracks, including phosphatidylserine, vitamin C, and zinc.

Tip #5—Lower excess water weight: Water retention can hide defined abdominal muscles. It is usually caused by excess sodium intake. Foods that are high in sodium include canned tuna, gravies, sauces, and breads. It is very important to maintain a 3:1 ratio of potassium-to-sodium for optimal water balance. Foods that are high in potassium include bananas and dates. Also, dandelion root is a powerful water-balancing herb that can help support the loss of excess body water, tighten the skin, and better define the abs.

Tip #6—Lose the booze: A study published in the *Journal of Advanced Nutrition and Human Metabolism* found that lipids (fats) accumulate in most tissues in which ethanol is metabolized. Alcohol seems to not only cause more fat storage but also lowers fat metabolism. Other research found that when comparing non-drinkers to recreational drinkers, the alcohol consumers had two to three times the number of abdominal fat deposits. If you want to have lean abs, it is best to put the alcohol back on the shelf and leave it there.

Tip #7—Manage estrogen levels: Estrogen is one of the body's most powerful fat-storage hormones. For men, managing estrogen levels can help limit fat storage in the abdominal region. Higher estrogen levels in men can cause abdominal fat storage, bloating, and fatigue. Make sure you don't have any mineral deficiencies, such as calcium or zinc, as these may be linked to elevated levels of estrogen. Drinking green tea and eating flaxseeds may help to lower estrogen levels as well.

the contest. If the peak day is Saturday, then take two capsules (500 milligrams (mg) per capsule) of dandelion root three times daily starting on Wednesday. On Saturday, take just two capsules first thing in the morning with a sip of water. You can also take 200 mg of caffeine two times daily starting Thursday before a Saturday peak day to further increase water depletion, as caffeine has mild diuretic properties.

You need to limit sodium intake to around 1,000 mg daily during this last week before peaking. This will help lower water retention and allow for your muscles to look lean. However, lowering sodium intake too much may stimulate the hormone aldosterone, which can actually cause you to retain more

Carbohydrate Depleting and Loading

Carbohydrate depleting and loading has been used by bodybuilders for decades and it is even employed by endurance athletes before a big race. The idea behind this technique is that by depleting carbohydrate stores, the body can allow more carbs to be stored in muscle tissue (by carb loading) than if depletion didn't take place. This is known as glycogen supercompensation. This is a fact, proven by research, but the process is very tricky. Many people try to use this technique and it actually backfires on them causing greater water retention (what bodybuilders call "spillover").

I recommend a fairly simple way to maximize this process, especially in phase 2 of the Six-Pack Diet Plan. Starting six days before a contest, try depleting carbohydrates for four days by consuming no more than 50 grams (g) of carbohydrates per day (preferably limiting their consumption to early in the day). This would be equivalent to a medium sweet potato or one bowl of multigrain oatmeal. Make sure the carbohydrate you consume is complex and low glycemic (that is, it elicits a low blood-sugar response). Make up the calorie deficit by consuming extra protein at this time. This depleting phase will increase glycogen synthase activity (the enzyme that helps make glycogen, thereby increasing stored carbohydrates in muscle tissue) and prime your body for glycogen supercompensation.

Training during this time should consist of heavy, explosive (concentric) movements for low repetitions. This will really deplete your glycogen levels. Glucagon (a blood sugar–controlling hormone) levels will start rising at this point to help maintain blood sugar levels. You may also start to feel lethargic as a result.

water. So, it is very important to restrict sodium intake to no less than 500 mg during the last 24 hours before a contest, since it takes twelve to twenty-four hours for aldosterone to "kick in" as a result of sodium depletion.

It is a good idea to take extra potassium about five days before a contest to increase the potassium-to-sodium ratio, thereby allowing optimal water balance and less intercellular water retention. Take 200 mg of potassium citrate two to three times daily with meals, starting five days before the contest.

All dairy products should be eliminated from the diet this last week as they tend to cause water retention in most people. Also, eliminate meal-

---

If the competition is on Saturday, the first day of carbohydrate depletion should be the Sunday before and the last day of carbohydrate depletion the Wednesday before. Start carbohydrate loading on Thursday and continue until the competition. Consume around 200–300 g of carbohydrates depending on body weight (generally, this is about 1.5 grams per pound of body weight) on both Thursday and Friday, consisting of high-glycemic carbs such as white rice, white potatoes, and rice cakes. Consume these carbs with the first four meals of the day and then have only fibrous carbs for the last two meals.

Use insulin-mimicking supplements with each meal during carbohydrate loading to better store the carbs in muscle tissue. Take vanadyl sulfate (40 mg); alpha-lipoic acid (100 mg); chromium polynicotinate (200 micrograms (mcg); D-pinitol (25 mg); and corosolic acid (12 mg) with each carbohydrate-containing meal during the carb-loading days. Also, take L-glutamine (5 g) with two of these meals to further enhance glycogen storage and cell volumization.

For maximum results, it is important not to weight train during carbohydrate loading. I recommend that your last cardio session be on Thursday morning if the event is on a Saturday. During the two days of carb-loading, another trick to harden up the muscles is to flex about thirty minutes after each carbohydrate-containing meal. You can do this anywhere: just tighten up your arms, chest, back, abs, and legs for about twenty seconds (not all at the same time, of course). You should actually pose every night for about thirty minutes in front of a mirror during the last week before a competition. This will be especially difficult during carbohydrate depleting, but it will help tighten the muscles and allow you to arrive in top shape.

replacement powders and protein shakes and replace them with food sources of protein (orange roughy, low-sodium tuna, and chicken breast). Again, many of these MRP formulas contain too much sodium and may cause unnecessary water retention. (Every little bit can make a difference in your physique during this critical time.)

The Big Day

You want to consume at least three protein and carbohydrate meals (for example, low-sodium tuna and one cup of cooked white rice) before the contest. The last full meal, about two hours before the contest, should consist of 8 ounces of lean sirloin steak and a medium baked potato (to help fill out the muscles). Make sure to take potassium citrate (200 mg) and all the insulin-mimicking supplements recommended earlier with each of your meals on this day. Remember to only sip water as needed and try to make as many trips to the bathroom as possible. (You've got to get that water out.) About forty-five minutes before the contest, consume the following supplements and foods (supplements first):

- L-arginine, 5 g

- Niacin, 100–200 mg

- Alpha-lipoic acid, 200 mg

- Vanadyl sulfate, 45 mg

- D-pinitol, 50 mg

- Chromium polynicotinate, 200 mcg

- Corosolic acid, 24 mg

- One or two large handfuls of raisins or other high-glycemic, sugary snack (to spike insulin levels and increase muscle pump)

- 1 tablespoon of natural peanut butter (the fat can help fill out the muscles)

Make sure you are warmed up beforehand: you can wear a sweatshirt or just break a slight sweat. About thirty minutes after consuming the foods and supplements, start pumping up by doing two sets of fifteen push-ups, two sets of bicep curls, one set of side laterals, two sets of abdominal crunches, and one set of pull-ups to the front. Do not pump up your legs as this takes blood away from your upper body and obscures the cuts in your legs as well. Pose hard for a few minutes right before the contest or photo shoot. Continue eating raisins every thirty minutes to an hour during the shoot or event as well.

Following phase 2 should allow you to get in top shape after following phase 1 of the Six-Pack Diet Plan. After this, you're ready to go on to phase 3 of the plan—the maintenance phase.

PHASE 3: SIX-PACK DIET MAINTENANCE

Once you've reached your fat-loss goal and the lean muscle mass you desire, then it is time to maintain these results without getting burned out. Remember, the Six-Pack Diet Plan is a lifestyle, not a quick fix. On the maintenance phase, the macronutrient ratios and calories will differ from phase 1 and cardiovascular work will be decreased to two days a week, but the overall program is similar.

STEP 1

Figure out caloric intake and daily nutrients. Multiply your body weight by twelve calories to determine how many calories need to be consumed daily at a ratio of 40 percent protein, 45 percent carbohydrates, and 15 percent essential fats. Here's how it breaks down:

Total Calories:

200 (pounds) $\times$ 12 calories = consume 2,400 calories daily

Protein:

40 percent protein = 2,400 $\times$ 0.40 = 960 total calories from protein daily

960 calories of protein $\div$ 4 calories per gram of protein = 240 g protein daily

Carbohydrates:

45 percent carbohydrates = 2,400 $\times$ 0.45 = 1,080 total calories from carbohydrates

1,080 calories of carbohydrates $\div$ 4 calories per gram of carbohydrates = 270 g carbs daily

TIP: Remember to consume a good portion of these carbs first thing in the morning and after a hard workout.

Fat:

15 percent fat = $2,400 \times 0.15$ = 360 total calories from fat daily

360 calories of fat $\div$ 9 calories per gram of fat = 40 g essential fats daily

DAILY CALORIE BREAKDOWN-MAINTENANCE PHASE				
Bodyweight (lbs)	Total Daily Calories	Protein (grams)	Carbohydrates (grams)	Fat (grams)
100	1,200	120	135	20
120	1,440	144	162	24
140	1,680	168	189	28
160	1,920	192	216	32
180	2,160	216	243	36
200	2,400	240	270	40
220	2,640	264	297	44
240	2,880	288	324	48
260	3,120	312	351	52
280	3,360	336	378	56
300	3,600	360	405	60

STEP 2

Divide up your meals so that a majority of your carbohydrates are consumed in the first meal of the day and the meal right after training. Eat six small meals daily. This helps increase the thermogenic effect of foods and modulates insulin levels to discourage fat storage. Use meal-replacement powders and protein bars for convenience. (See Chapter 2.)

STEP 3

Watch your sodium intake as this can make you retain water and hide your abdominal definition. High-sodium foods include gravies, sauces, soups, breads, canned meats, and condiments like ketchup.

STEP 4

Drink at least one gallon of water daily.

STEP 5

Have a reward meal containing high protein, simple carbohydrates, and fats. Examples include a cheese omelet with blueberry pancakes or a sirloin steak with mashed potatoes and dessert. Eat this meal slowly and only have it once per week, if you have earned it. Consider it your reward for adhering strictly to the plan during the week.

STEP 6

Take the same supplements as in phase 1, except use no thermogenic products or stimulant products during this phase.

STEP 7

The resistance training routine is the same as in phase 1. Cardio is done only twice per week—one day of sprints, then one day of moderately-paced, longer-duration cardio, such as walking on a treadmill for thirty-five minutes.

SIX-PACK DIET MAINTENANCE BASICS

- Be consistent. It is important to follow this plan uninterrupted for several months. The Six-Pack Diet Plan is based on long-term, *permanent* change, not on a quick-fix fad.

- Drink plenty of water. Try consuming at least one gallon of water *daily*, especially if strenuously exercising.

- Eat frequent, small meals daily. Eating six to eight smaller meals throughout the day can be highly beneficial.

- Don't be "carbo-phobic." Eat the right type of carbohydrates (complex rather than simple) in moderate amounts and at the key times as discussed in Chapter 2.

- Plan your meals ahead of time. Cook your meals for the week on Sunday and store them in the fridge or freezer. Keep protein shakes and bars with you at all times.

- Eat mixed meals. Every meal (except the last few of the day) should consist of protein and carbohydrates/fiber.

- Make "better bad choices." For example, instead of regular potato chips, have the baked chips (which are lower in fat). Or instead of regular ice cream, have non-fat frozen yogurt. Try the low- or nonfat versions of salad dressings and dairy products instead of the high-fat versions.

- Make a commitment and stick to the program by setting realistic goals. You must have a fitness goal before starting this program. Setting goals puts positive pressure on you to achieve fitness success. Whether it's losing four dress sizes or eliminating twenty pounds of fat, you need to determine what your end result will be. Not having a goal is like getting in your car and driving without having a destination.

- Execute. Only you can determine your own success. Ultimately, you are responsible for succeeding or failing on the program.

Now you have leading-edge information that can change your body permanently. By sticking to the Six-Pack Diet Plan, you can be on your way to lean abs and a strong muscular body. Set a goal and then use this program to get the results you desire. The Six-Pack Diet Plan lifestyle enables long-term fat loss and will make your abs leaner than ever.

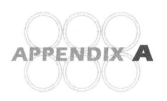

APPENDIX A

Sample Six-Pack Meal Plans

SIX-PACK MEAL PLAN ~1,500 CALORIES

Meal 1

Six egg whites, boiled with pepper and 1 teaspoon flaxseed oil

$\frac{1}{2}$ cup cooked multi-grain oatmeal with 1 teaspoon cinnamon

Fish oil capsules (2 g)

Opti-Pack by Super Nutrition (1 packet)

Hydroxycut or Lean Fire (one serving)

Guggulsterones (25 mg)

Meal 2 (Post-workout)

One packet Eat-Smart MRP or Low-Carb Lean Body
with 16 ounces water

1 tablespoon honey

Three small dates

L-arginine (3 g)

Alpha-lipoic acid (200 mg)

D-pinitol (100 mg)

Rhodiola rosea (100 mg)

AbGONE (two softgels)

Meal 3

5 ounces chicken breast, cooked with 1 teaspoon olive oil

$\frac{1}{2}$ cup cooked brown rice

One large serving garden salad

One cup green tea

Hydroxycut or Lean Fire (one serving)

Alpha-lipoic acid (100 mg)

D-pinitol (100 mg)

Meal 4

3 ounces baked mahi mahi

$\frac{1}{2}$ sweet potato

Guggulsterones (25 mg)

Meal 5

3 ounces baked mahi mahi

$\frac{1}{2}$ sweet potato

AbGONE (two softgels)

Meal 6

5 ounces orange roughy fish (baked plain)

1 cup broccoli and cauliflower

Guggulsterones (25 mg)

Meal 7

Four egg whites, boiled with pepper

One small serving salad containing mainly lettuce

Meal 8

One serving protein powder (containing both whey and casein) with 8 ounces water

L-glutamine (5 g)

Phosphatidylserine (400 mg)

Rhodiola rosea (100 mg)

Alpha GPC (250 mg)

Opti-Pack by Super Nutrition (one pack)

SIX-PACK MEAL PLAN ~2,000 CALORIES

Meal 1

Eight egg whites, boiled with pepper and 1 teaspoon flaxseed oil

1 cup cooked multi-grain oatmeal with 1 teaspoon cinnamon

Fish oil capsules (2 g)

Opti-Pack by Super Nutrition (one pack)

Hydroxycut or Lean Fire (one serving)

Guggulsterones (25 mg)

Meal 2 (Post-workout)

One packet MRP (such as Micellean Bioactive Superfood)
with 8 ounces water or apple juice, and 1 teaspoon honey

L-arginine (5 g)

Alpha-lipoic acid (200 mg)

D-pinitol (100 mg)

Rhodiola rosea (200 mg)

AbGONE (two softgels)

Meal 3

6 ounces chicken breast, cooked with one teaspoon olive oil

1 cup cooked brown rice

1 cup broccoli and cauliflower

One cup green tea

Hydroxycut or Lean Fire (one serving)

Alpha-lipoic acid (100 mg)

D-pinitol (100 mg)

Meal 4

$\frac{1}{2}$ can low-sodium tuna

$\frac{1}{2}$ sweet potato

AbGONE (two softgels)

Guggulsterones (25 mg)

Meal 5

$^1/_2$ can low-sodium tuna

$^1/_2$ sweet potato

AbGONE (2 softgels)

Meal 6

8 ounces orange roughy fish (baked plain)

1 large cup broccoli and cauliflower

Guggulsterones (25 mg)

Meal 7

1 serving protein powder (containing both whey and casein)
with 8 ounces water

Meal 8

Six egg whites, boiled with pepper

One small serving salad containing mainly lettuce

L-glutamine (5 g)

Phosphatidylserine (400 mg)

Rhodiola rosea (100 mg)

Alpha GPC (250 mg)

Opti-Pack by Super Nutrition (one pack)

ZMA-T™ (one serving)

SIX-PACK MEAL PLAN ~2,500 CALORIES

Meal 1

Ten egg whites, boiled with pepper and 1 teaspoon flaxseed oil

1 cup cooked multi-grain oatmeal with 1 teaspoon cinnamon

Fish oil capsules (2 g)

MegaMen by GNC (recommended serving)

Hydroxycut or Redline (one serving)

Guggulsterones (25 mg)

Meal 2 (Post-workout)

One packet MRP (such as Micellean Bioactive Superfood)
with 16 ounces water and 1 tablespoon honey

$\frac{1}{2}$ cup raisins

L-arginine (5 g)

Alpha-lipoic acid (200 mg)

D-pinitol (100 mg)

Rhodiola rosea (200 mg)

AbGONE (two softgels)

Meal 3

8 ounces lean sirloin steak, cooked with 1 teaspoon olive oil

1 cup cooked brown rice

One large serving garden salad

One cup green tea

Hydroxycut or Redline (one serving)

Alpha-lipoic acid (100 mg)

D-pinitol (100 mg)

Meal 4

4 ounces chicken breast

$1/2$ sweet potato

AbGONE (two softgels)

Guggulsterones (25 mg)

Meal 5

4 ounces chicken breast

$1/2$ sweet potato

AbGONE (two softgels)

Meal 6

8 ounces salmon (baked plain)

1 large cup broccoli and cauliflower

Guggulsterones (25 mg)

Meal 7

Low-carb protein bar (such as Keto Bar or Nitro-Tech bar)

Meal 8

Two servings protein powder (containing both whey and casein) with 8 ounces water

L-glutamine (5 g)

Phosphatidylserine (400 mg)

Rhodiola rosea (100 mg)

Alpha GPC (250 mg)

MegaMen by GNC (recommended serving)

ZMA-T (one serving)

For personalized Six-Pack meal plans, please contact:
Rehan Jalali
Tel: 310-858-5583
E-mail: rehan@tsrf.com

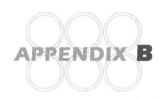

APPENDIX **B**

Information and Supplement Resources

BOOKS

ABSolution: The Practical Solution for Building Your Best Abs by Shawn Phillips (Golden, CO: High Point Media, 2002).
A comprehensive book on abdominal training; recommended for Six-Pack Dieters. Shawn Phillips also has a website with additional ab training tips: www.BestAbs.com

The Men's Health Book of Muscle by Lou Schuler and Ian King (Emmaus, PA: Rodale, 2003).
A detailed book on exercises and muscle groups; very comprehensive, yet easy to read.

MAGAZINES

Physical Magazine
11050 Santa Monica Blvd.,
  3rd Floor
Los Angeles, CA 90025
Website: www.physicalmag.com
A sports nutrition magazine with easy-to-read and detailed information on fitness, health, nutrition, supplements, and exercise.

Real SOLUTIONS Magazine
P.O. Box 17172
Golden, CO 80402
Tel: 866-688-7679

Fax: 303-215-1386
Website: www.realsolutionsmag.com
A fitness magazine that provides the latest information on nutrition, training, and supplements.

Men's Fitness Magazine
One Park Ave., 10th Floor
New York, NY 10016
Website: www.mensfitness.com
A fitness magazine with solid and useful information.

EXPERTS

Vince Andrich
Gerstner and Associates Inc.
E-mail: vandrich@gerstnerinc.com

Vince is one of the most experienced individuals in nutrition, sports supplements, and training. He is also a leading fitness author.

Gunnar Peterson, CSCS
Developer of Core Secrets
www.coresecrets.com

Gunnar is one of the top trainers in the world. He trains Hollywood celebrities, professional athletes, and everyday people.

Karlis Ullis, M.D.
1807 Wilshire Blvd.
Santa Monica, CA 90403
Tel: 310-829-1990
Fax: 310-829-5134

Dr. Ullis is one of the top anti-aging/hormone experts in the world. He is author of The Hormone Revolution Weight Loss Plan (New York: Avery, 2003) and Super T (New York: Fireside/Simon & Schuster, 1999).

FURTHER INFORMATION

The Supplement Research Foundation
468 N. Camden Drive
Suite 200, Second Floor
Beverly Hills, CA 90210
Tel: 310-858-5583
Fax: 310-858-5500
Website: www.tsrf.com

This organization (founded by Rehan Jalali) provides cutting-edge, research-based information about dietary supplements, nutrition, and fitness in general.

U.S.D.A. Nutrient Data Laboratory
Agricultural Research Service/
 Beltsville Human Nutrition
 Research Center
10300 Baltimore Avenue

Building 005, Room 107,
 BARC-West
Beltsville, MD 20705-2350
Tel: 301-504-0630
Fax: 301-504-0632
Website: www.nal.usda.gov/fnic/
 foodcomp

Nutrition profiles for thousands of foods provided by the United States government's Agricultural Research Service. The website has a great search function that allows you to find comprehensive nutrient profiles for many foods.

NutritionData.com
Website: www.nutritiondata.com

Another website that provides a database of virtually every nutrient contained in most foods. It is great for counting calories and macronutrient contents of foods.

SUPPLEMENT SOURCES

Biotech Research
7800 Whipple Avenue NW
Canton, Oh 44767
Tel: 800-764-0009
Website: www.abgone.com

Makers of AbGONE™, a dietary supplement containing conjugated linoleic acid (CLA) and nutrients targeting abdominal fat.

EAS
555 Corporate Circle
Golden, CO 80401
Tel: 800-297-9776
Fax: 303-279-6465
Website: www.eas.com

Leading sports supplement company with products like Myoplex Deluxe™.

FSI Nutrition
14920 Grover Street
Omaha, NE 68144
Tel: 402-333-3532

Source of Phosphate Edge™ and leaders in effervescent technology.

Global Nutrition Sciences Inc.
Arvada, CO 80004
Tel: 800-595-4670
Website: www.global-nutrition. com

A supplement resource providing leading-edge products from fat burners to energy boosters to nutrition-balancing shakes and bars.

Instone Nutrition
University Research Park
5251 California, Suite 150
Irvine, CA 92612
Tel: 949-854-1600

A company founded by actor Sylvester Stallone and a source of the thermogenic supplement Lean Fire. They also provide solid fitness information and additional active lifestyle products.

iSatori Technologies
15000 W. 6th Avenue,
  Suite 202
Golden, CO 80401
Tel: 866-688-7679
Fax: 303-215-1386
Website: www.leansystem7.com

Provider of the scientifically based Lean System 7™ fat-loss product, delicious Eat-Smart MRP, and the creatine product Meta-Cel™.

MHP (Maximum Human Performance)
1376 Pompton Avenue
Cedar Grove, NJ 07009
Tel: 888-783-8844
Website: www.maxperformance. com

This sports nutrition company provides leading-edge products as well as quality fitness information.

Muscle-Link

1701 Ives Avenue
Oxnard, CA 93033
Tel: 800-570-4766

Source of Cort-Bloc™, GH STAK™, and ZMA-T™; an honest and reputable company.

MuscleTech Research and Development

Mississauga, ON, Canada L6W 4S6
Tel: 877-443-4074
Website: www.muscletech.com

A quality sports nutrition company providing numerous products that fit into the Six-Pack Diet Plan, including Hydroxycut® and Nitro-Tech™.

SAN

716 N. Ventura Road #431
Oxnard, CA 93030
Tel: 888-519-9300

Source of T3, containing guggulipids, and other cutting-edge supplements.

Syntrax

P.O Box 1593
Cape Girardeau, MO 63702
Tel: 888-321-2348

Source of Guggulbolic, containing guggulipids.

VPX

Davie, FL 33314
Tel: 800-954-7904
Website: www.vpxsports.com

Provider of highly advanced supplements, including Redline and Micellean Bioactive Superfood, a top meal-replacement powder.

Selected References

Chapter 1: How the Body Burns Fat

Brillon, D.J., B. Zheng, R.G. Campbell, et al. "Effect of Cortisol on Energy Expenditure and Amino Acid Metabolism in Humans." *Am J Physiol* 268:3 Part 1 (1995): E501–513.

Broca, C., R. Gross, P. Petit, et al. "4-Hydroxyisoleucine: Experimental Evidence of Its Insulinotropic and Antidiabetic Properties." *Am J Physiol* 277:4 Part 1 (1999): E617–E623.

Chrousos, G., et al. "CRH, Stress and Depression: An Etiological Approach." Conference on Cortisol and Anti-Cortisols, Las Vegas, NV, 1997.

Del Mar Gonzalez-Barroso, M., D. Ricquier, and A.M. Cassard-Doulcier. "The Human Uncoupling Protein-1 Gene (UCP1): Present Status and Perspectives in Obesity Research." *Obes Rev* 1:2 (2000): 61–72.

Epel, E., R. Lapidus, B. McEwen, and K. Brownell. "Stress May Add Bite to Appetite in Women: A Laboratory Study of Stress-induced Cortisol and Eating Behavior." *Psychoneuroendocrinology* 26:1 (2001): 37–49.

Epel, E.E., A.E. Moyer, C.D. Martin, et al. "Stress-induced Cortisol, Mood, and Fat Distribution in Men." *Obes Res* 7:1 (1999): 9–15.

Epel, E.S., B. McEwen, T. Seeman, et al. "Stress and Body Shape: Stress-induced Cortisol Secretion is Consistently Greater Among Women with Central Fat." *Psychosomatic Med* 62:5 (2000): 623–632.

Fawcett, J.P., S.J. Farquhar, R.J. Walker, et al. "The Effect of Oral Vanadyl Sulfate on Body Composition and Performance in Weight-training Athletes." *Int J Sport Nutr* 6:4 (1996): 382–390.

Friedman, J.E., P.D. Neufer, and G.L. Dohm. "Regulation of Glycogen Resynthesis Following Exercise. Dietary Considerations." *Sports Med* 11:4 (1991): 232–243.

Grant, K.E., R.M. Chandler, A.L. Castle, et al. "Chromium and Exercise Training: Effect on Obese Women." *Med Sci Sports Exerc* 29 (1997): 992–998.

Griffin, J., and S. Ojeda. *Textbook of Endocrine Physiology,* 3rd ed. New York: Oxford University Press, 1996.

Hofbauer, K.G. "Molecular Pathways to Obesity." *Int J Obes Relat Metab Disord* 26:Suppl 2 (2002): S18–S27.

Hofman, L.F. "Human Saliva as a Diagnostic Specimen." *J Nutr* 131:5 (2001): 1621S–1625S.

Ikeda, Y. "The Clinical Study on the Water Extract of Leaves of *Lagerstroemia speciosa L* for Mild Cases of Diabetes Mellitus." Tokyo: Jikeikai University, 1998 (pilot study data).

Jamieson, J., L. Dorman, and V. Marriot. *Growth Hormone: Reversing Human Aging Naturally.* East Canaan, CT: Safe Goods, 1997.

Johnston, C.S., C.S. Day, and P.D. Swan. "Postprandial Thermogenesis is Increased 100% on a High-protein, Low-fat Diet versus a High-carbohydrate, Low-fat Diet in Healthy, Young Women." *J Am Coll Nutr* 21:1 (2002): 55–61.

Kanaley, J., J.Y. Weltman, K.S. Pieper, et al. "Cortisol and Growth Hormone Responses to Exercise at Different Times of the Day." *J Clin Endocrinol Metab* 86:6 (2001): 2881–2889.

Kelley, D., et al. "Energy Restriction and Immunocompetence in Overweight Women." *Nutrition Research* 18:2 (1998): 159–169.

Khalil, D.A., E.A. Lucas, S. Juma, et al. "Soy Protein Supplementation Increases Serum Insulin-like Growth Factor-I in Young and Old Men but Does Not Affect Markers of Bone Metabolism." *J Nutr* 132:9 (2002): 2605–2608.

Klip, A., T. Ramal, D.A. Young, et al. "Insulin-induced Translocation of Glucose Transporters in Rat Hindlimb Muscles." *FEBS Lett* 224:1 (1987): 224–230.

LeBlanc, J., I. Mercier, and A. Nadeau. "Components of Postprandial Thermogenesis in Relation to Meal Frequency in Humans." *Can J Physiol Pharmacol* 71:12 (1993): 879–883.

Medvedev, L.N., and E.I. Elsukova. "Brown Fat Tissue in Humans." *Usp Fiziol Nauk* 33:2 (2002): 17–29.

Narayanan, C. "Pinitol—A New Anti-Diabetic Compound From the Leaves of Bougainvillea." *Current Science* 56:3 (1987): 139–141.

Newsholme, E.A., and A.R. Leech. *Biochemistry for the Medical Sciences.* New York: John Wiley & Sons, 1984, 38-42, 312-30, 444–454.

Ng, T.B., C.M. Wong, W.W. Li, and H.W. Yeung. "Insulin-like Molecules in *Momordica charantia* Seeds." *J Ethnopharmacol* 15:1 (1986): 107–117.

Packer, L. "Antioxidant Properties of Lipoic Acid and Its Therapeutic Effects in Prevention of Diabetes Complications and Cataracts." *Annals NY Acad Sci* 738 (1994): 257–264.

Rizza, R.A., L.J. Mandarino, and J.E. Gerich. "Cortisol-induced Insulin Resistance in Man: Impaired Suppression of Glucose Production and Stimulation of Glucose Utilization Due to a Postreceptor Detect of Insulin Action." *J Clin Endocrinol Metab* 54:1 (1982): 131–138.

Rodnick, K.J., E.J. Henriksen, D.E. James, et al. "Exercise Training, Glucose Transporters, and Glucose Transport in Rat Skeletal Muscles." *Am J Physiol* 262:1 (1992): C9–C14.

Simmons, P.S., J.M. Miles, J.E. Gerich, et al. "Increased Proteolysis: An Effect of Increases in Plasma Cortisol Within the Physiologic Range." *J Clin Invest* 73:2 (1984): 412–420.

Ullis, Karlis, M.D. From an interview in *BodyModern Magazine* 1:1 (2003). Available on the Internet. www.prolab.com.

Wallberg-Henriksson, H., S.H. Constable, D.A. Young, et al. "Glucose Transport Into Rat Skeletal Muscle: Interaction Between Exercise and Insulin." *J Appl Physiol* 65:2 (1998): 909–913.

Welihinda, J., E.H. Karunanayake, M.H. Sheriff, et al. "Effect of *Momordica charantia* on the Glucose Tolerance in Maturity Onset Diabetes." *J Ethnopharmacol* 17:3 (1986): 277–282.

Chapter 2: The Six-Pack Eating Plan

Arnold, L.M., M.J. Ball, A.W. Duncan, et al. "Effect of Isoenergetic Intake of Three or Nine Meals on Plasma Lipoproteins and Glucose Metabolism." *Am J Clin Nutr* 57:3 (1993): 446–451.

Bloomer, R.J., G.A. Sforzo, and B.A. Keller. "Effects of Meal Form and Composition on Plasma Testosterone, Cortisol, and Insulin Following Resistance Exercise." *Int J Sport Nutr Exerc Metab* 10:4 (2000): 415–424.

Borkman, M., L.H. Storlien, D.A. Pan, et al. "The Relationship Between Insulin Sensitivity and the Fatty Acid Composition of Skeletal-muscle Phospholipids." *N Engl J Med* 328:4 (1993): 238–244.

Brilla, L.R., and V. Conte. "Effects of Zinc-magnesium Formulation Increases Anabolic Hormones and Strength in Athletes." *Med Sci Sports Exerc* 31:5 (1999): 483.

Broca, C., R. Gross, P. Petit, et al. "4-Hydroxyisoleucine: Experimental Evidence of Its Insulinotropic and Antidiabetic Properties." *Am J Physiol* 277:4 Part 1 (1999): E617–E623.

D'Adamo, P. "Larch arabinogalactan." *J Naturopath Med* 6 (1996): 33–37.

De Combarieu, E., N. Fuzzati, M. Lovati, et al. "Furostanol Saponins from *Tribulus terrestris*." *Fitoterapia* 74:6 (2003): 583–591.

Demling, R.H., and L. DeSanti. "Effect of a Hypocaloric Diet, Increased Protein Intake and Resistance Training on Lean Mass Gains and Fat Mass Loss in Overweight Police Officers." *Ann Nutr Metab* 44:1 (2000): 21–29.

Desroches, S., et al. "Effects of Dietary Conjugated Linoleic Acid on Plasma Lipoproteins and Body Composition in Obese Men." *Obesity Res* 9 Suppl 3 (2001): 87S–87S.

Doi, T., T. Matsuo, M. Sugawara, et al. "New Approach for Weight Reduction by a Combination of Diet, Light Resistance Exercise and the Timing of Ingesting a Protein Supplement." *Asia Pacific J Clin Nutr* 10:3 (2001): 226–232.

Dorgan, J., J.T. Judd, C. Longcope, et al. "Effects of Dietary Fat and Fiber on Plasma and Urine Androgens and Estrogens in Men: A Controlled Feeding Study." *Am J Clin Nutr* 64:6 (1996): 850–855.

Dray, F., B. Kouznetzova, D. Harris, et al. "Role of Prostaglandins on Growth Hormone Secretion: PGE2, a Physiological Stimulator." *Adv Prostaglandin Thromboxane Res* 8 (1980): 1321–1328.

Erasmus, U. *Fats That Heal, Fats That Kill.* Burnaby, BC, Canada: Alive Books, 1993.

Esmarck, B., J.L. Andersen, S. Olsen, et al. "Timing of Postexercise Protein Intake is Important for Muscle Hypertrophy with Resistance Training in Elderly Humans." *J Physiol* 15:535 Part 1 (2001): 301–311.

Forsling, M.L., M.J. Wheeler, and A.J. Williams. "The Effect of Melatonin Administration on Pituitary Hormone Secretion in Man." *Clin Endocrinol* (Oxford) 51:5 (1999): 637–642.

Garg, M.L., A. Wierzbicki, M. Keelan, et al. "Fish Oil Prevents Change in Arachidonic Acid and Cholesterol Content in Rat Caused by Dietary Cholesterol." *Lipids* 24:4 (1989): 266–270.

Ghigo, E., E. Arvat, and F. Camanni. "Orally Active Growth Hormone Secretagogues: State of the Art and Clinical Perspectives." *Ann Med* 30:2 (1998): 159–168.

Griffiths, R.D. "Glutamine: Establishing Clinical Indications." *Curr Opin Clin Nutr Metab Care* 2:2 (1999): 177–182.

Groff, J., S. Gropper, and S. Hunt. *Advanced Nutrition and Human Metabolism,* 2nd ed. St. Paul, MN: West, 1995.

Ivy, J.L. "Dietary Strategies to Promote Glycogen Synthesis After Exercise." *Can J Appl Physiol* 26 (2001): S236–S245.

Kelly, G.S. "*Rhodiola rosea:* A Possible Plant Adaptogen." *Altern Med Rev* 6:3 (2001): 293–302.

LeBlanc, J., I. Mercier, and A. Nadeau. "Components of Postprandial Thermogenesis in Relation to Meal Frequency in Humans." *Can J Physiol Pharmacol* 71:12 (1993): 879–883.

Liu, Z., L.A. Jahn, W. Long, et al. "Branched Chain Amino Acids Activate Messenger Ribonucleic Acid Translation Regulatory Proteins in Human Skeletal Muscle, and Glucocorticoids Blunt This Action." *J Clin Endocrinol Metab* 86:5 (2001): 2136–2143.

Monteleone, P., L. Beinat, C. Tanzillo, et al. "Effects of Phosphatidylserine on the Neuroendocrine Responses to Physical Stress in Humans." *Neuroendocrinol* 52:3 (1990): 243–248.

Montner, P., D.M. Stark, M.L. Riedesel, et al. "Pre-exercise Glycerol Hydration Improves Cycling Endurance Time." *Int J Sports Med* 17:1 (1996): 27–33.

Peters, E.M., R. Anderson, D.C. Nieman, et al. "Vitamin C Supplementation Attenuates the Increases in Circulating Cortisol, Adrenaline and Anti-inflammatory Polypeptides Following Ultramarathon Running." *Int J Sports Med* 22:7 (2001): 537–543.

Potter, S.M. "Overview of Proposed Mechanisms for the Hypocholesterolemic Effect of Soy." *J Nutr* 125:3 Suppl (1995): 606S–611S.

Robergs, R., and S. Griffin. "Glycerol. Biochemistry, Pharmacokinetics and Clinical and Practical Applications." *Sports Med* 26:3 (1998): 145–167.

Van Hall, G., W.H. Saris, P.A. van de Schoor, et al. "The Effect of Free Glutamine and Peptide Ingestion on the Rate of Muscle Glycogen Resynthesis in Man." *Int J Sports Med* 21:1 (2000): 25–30.

Warner, J., et al. "Combined Effects of Aerobic Exercise and Omega-3 Fatty-acids on Plasma Lipids in Hyperlipidemic Subjects." *Clin Res* 34:2 (1986): 806A.

Welbourne, T.C. "Increased Plasma Bicarbonate and Growth Hormone After an Oral Glutamine Load." *Am J Clin Nutr* 61:5 (1995): 1058–1061.

Wenos, D.L., and H.K. Amato. "Weight Cycling Alters Muscular Strength and Endurance, Ratings of Perceived Exertion, and Total Body Water in College Wrestlers." *Percept Motor Skills* 87:3 Part 1 (1998): 975–978.

Chapter 3: Fat-Loss Supplements

Agarwal, R.C., S.P. Singh, R.K. Saran, et al. "Clinical Trials of Gugulipid—A New Hypolipidemic Agent of Plant Origin in Primary Hyperlipidemia." *Indian J Med Res* 84 (1986): 626–634.

Andersen, T., and J. Fogh. "Weight Loss and Delayed Gastric Emptying Following a South American Herbal Preparation in Overweight Patients." *J Hum Nutr Diet* 14:3 (2001): 243–250.

Anderson, M.E., C.R. Bruce, S.F. Fraser, et al. "Enhancement of 2000-m Rowing Performance After Caffeine Ingestion." *Med Sci Sports Exerc* 32:11 (2000): 1958–1963.

Avraham, Y., S. Hao, S. Mendelson, et al. "Tyrosine Improves Appetite, Cognition, and Exercise Tolerance in Activity Anorexia." *Med Sci Sports Exerc* 33:12 (2001): 2104–2110.

Belury, M.A., A. Mahon, and S. Banni. "The Conjugated Linoleic Acid (CLA) Isomer, t10c12-CLA, is Inversely Associated with Changes in Body Weight and Serum Leptin in Subjects with Type 2 Diabetes Mellitus." *J Nutr* 133:1 (2003): 257S–260S.

Bour, S., V. Visentin, D. Prevot, et al. "Moderate Weight-lowering Effect of Octopamine Treatment in Obese Zucker Rats." *J Physiol Biochem* 59:3 (2003): 175–182.

Colker, C., et al. "Effects of Citrus Aurantium Extract, Caffeine, and St. John's Wort on Body Fat Loss, Lipid Levels, and Mood States in Overweight Healthy Adults." *Curr Ther Res* 60:3 (1999): 145–153.

Desroches, S., et al. "Effects of Dietary Conjugated Linoleic Acid on Plasma Lipoproteins and Body Composition in Obese Men." *Obesity Res* 9 Suppl 3 (2001): 87S–87S.

Doherty, M. "The Effects of Caffeine on the Maximum Accumulated Oxygen Deficit and Short-term Running Performance." *Int J Sport Nutr* 8:2 (1998): 95–104.

Dulloo, A.G., C. Duret, D. Rohrer, et al. "Efficacy of a Green Tea Extract Rich in Catechin Polyphenols and Caffeine in Increasing 24-hour Energy Expenditure and Fat Oxidation in Humans." *Am J Clin Nutr* 70:6 (1999): 1040–1045.

Dulloo, A.G., J. Seydoux, L. Girardier, et al. "Green Tea and Thermogenesis: Interactions Between Catechin Polyphenols, Caffeine and Sympathetic Activity." *Int J Obes Relat Metab Disord* 24:2 (2000): 252–258.

Gaullier, J.M., G. Berven, H. Blankson, et al. "Clinical Trial Results Support a Preference for Using CLA Preparations Enriched with Two Isomers Rather than Four Isomers in Human Studies." *Lipids* 37:11 (2003): 1019–1025.

Gopal, K., R.K. Saran, S. Nityanand, et al. "Clinical Trial of Ethyl Acetate Extract of Gum Gugulu (Gugulipid) in Primary Hyperlipidemia." *J Assoc Physicians India* 34:4 (1986): 249–251.

Gorostiaga, E.M., C.A. Maurer, and J.P. Eclache. "Decrease in Respiratory Quotient During Exercise Following L-carnitine Supplementation." *Int J Sports Med* 10:3 (1989): 169–174.

Graham, T. "Caffeine and Exercise: Metabolism, Endurance, and Performance." *Sports Med* 31:11 (2001): 78580–7.

Graham, T. "Caffeine, Coffee, and Ephedrine: Impact on Exercise Performance and Metabolism." *Can J Appl Physiol* 26 Suppl (2001): S103–S119.

Griffin, J., and S. Ojeda. *Textbook of Endocrine Physiology* 3rd ed. New York: Oxford University Press, 1996.

Heymsfield, S.B., D.B. Allison, J.R. Vasselli, et al. "*Garcinia cambogia* (Hydroxycitric

Acid) as a Potential Antiobesity Agent: A Randomized Controlled Trial." *JAMA* 280:18 (1998): 1596–1600.

Kaciuba-Uscilko, H., K. Nazar, J. Chwalbinska-Moneta, et al. "Effect of Phosphate Supplementation on Metabolic and Neuroendocrine Responses to Exercise and Oral Glucose Load in Obese Women During Weight Reduction." *J Physiol Pharmacol* 44:4 (1993): 425–440.

Kalman, D., et al. "A Randomized, Double-Blind, Placebo Controlled Study of 3-Acetyl-7-Oxo-Dehydroepiandrosterone in Healthy Overweight Adults." *Curr Ther Res* 61:7 (2000): 435–442.

Kamphuis, M.M., M.P. Lejeune, W.H. Saris, et al. "The Effect of Conjugated Linoleic Acid Supplementation after Weight Loss on Body Weight Regain, Body Composition, and Resting Metabolic Rate in Overweight Subjects." *Int J Obes Relat Metab Disord* 27:7 (2003): 840–847.

Khajuria, A., U. Zutshi, and K.L. Bedi. "Permeability Characteristics of Piperine on Oral Absorption—An Active Alkaloid from Peppers and a Bioavailability Enhancer." *Indian J Exp Biol* 36:1 (1998): 46–50.

Laurenza, A., E.M. Sutkowski, and K.B. Seamon. "Forskolin: A Specific Stimulator of Adenylyl Cyclase or a Diterpene with Multiple Sites of Action?" *Trends Pharmacol Sci* 10:11 (1989): 442–447.

Lee, E.B., et al. "Pharmacological Study on Piperine." *Arch Pharmac Res* 7 (1984): 127–132.

McCarty, M. "Optimizing Exercise for Fat Loss." *Med Hypotheses* 44:5 (1995): 325–330.

Muller, D.M., H. Seim, W. Kiess, et al. "Effects of Oral L-carnitine Supplementation on In Vivo Long-chain Fatty Acid Oxidation in Healthy Adults." *Metabolism* 51:11 (2002): 1389–1391.

Mumford, G.K., S.M. Evans, B.J. Kaminski, et al. "Discriminative Stimulus and Subjective Effects of Theobromine and Caffeine in Humans." *Psychopharmacology* (Berlin) 115:1-2 (1994): 1–8.

Nazar, K., H. Kaciuba-Uscilko, J. Szczepanik, et al. "Phosphate Supplementation Prevents a Decrease of Triiodothyronine and Increases Resting Metabolic Rate During Low Energy Diet." *J Physiol Pharmacol* 47:2 (1996): 373–383.

Nehlig, A., and G. Debry. "Caffeine and Sports Activity." *Int J Sports Med* 15:5 (1994): 215–223.

Neri, D.F., D. Wiegmann, R.R. Stanny, et al. "The Effects of Tyrosine on Cognitive Performance During Extended Wakefulness." *Aviat Space Environ Med* 66:4 (1995): 313–319.

Nityanand, S., J.S. Srivastava, and O.P. Asthana. "Clinical Trials with Gugulipid. A New Hypolipidaemic Agent." *J Assoc Physicians India* 37:5 (1989): 323–328.

Pauly, D.F., and C.J. Pepine. "The Role of Carnitine in Myocardial Dysfunction." *Am J Kidney Dis* 41:4 Suppl 4 (2003): S35–S43.

Preuss, H.G., D. Bagchi, C.V.S. Rao, et al. "Effect of Hydroxycitric Acid on Weight Loss, Body Mass Index and Plasma Leptin Levels in Human Subjects." *FASEB Journal* 16 (2002): A1020, Abstract 742.16.

Racz-Kotilla, E., G. Racz, and A. Solomon. "The Action of *Taraxacum officinale* Extracts on the Body Weight and Diuresis of Laboratory Animals." *Planta Med* 26:3 (1974): 212–217.

Villani, R.G., J. Gannon, M. Self, et al. "L-Carnitine Supplementation Combined with Aerobic Training Does Not Promote Weight Loss in Moderately Obese Women." *Int J Sport Nutr Exerc Metab* 10:2 (2000): 199–207.

Volek, J.S., W.J. Kraemer, M.R. Rubin, et al. "L-Carnitine L-Tartrate Supplementation Favorably Affects Markers of Recovery From Exercise Stress." *Am J Physiol Endocrinol Metab* 282:2 (2002): E474–E482.

Watanabe, T., T. Kawada, and K. Iwai. "Effect of Capsaicin Pretreatment on Capsaicin-induced Catecholamine from the Adrenal Medulla in Rats." *Proc Soc Exp Biol Med* 187:3 (1988): 370–374.

Westerterp-Plantenga, M.S., and E.M. Kovacs. "The Effects of (-)-Hydroxycitrate on Energy Intake and Satiety in Overweight Humans." *Int J Obes Relat Metab Disord* 26:6 (2002): 870–872.

Yoshida, T., N. Sakane, T. Umekawa, et al. "Relationship Between Basal Metabolic Rate, Thermogenic Response to Caffeine, and Body Weight Loss Following Combined Low Calorie and Exercise Treatment in Obese Women." *Int J Obes Relat Metab Disord* 18:5 (1994): 345–350.

Yoshioka, M., S. St-Pierre, V. Drapeau, et al. "Effects of Red Pepper on Appetite and Energy Intake." *Br J Nutr* 82:2 (1999): 115–123.

Chapter 4: Hormone-Modifying Strategies

Anderson, J.W., N.J. Gustafson, C.A. Bryant, et al. "Dietary Fiber and Diabetes: A Comprehensive Review and Practical Application." *J Am Diet Assoc* 87:9 (1987): 1189–1197.

Argente, J., L.M. Garcia-Segura, J. Pozo, et al. "Growth Hormone-releasing Peptides: Clinical and Basic Aspects." *Horm Res* 46:4-5 (1996): 155–159.

Boden, G., X. Chen, J. Ruiz, et al. "Effects of Vanadyl Sulfate on Carbohydrate and Lipid Metabolism in Patients with Non-insulin-dependent Diabetes Mellitus." *Metabolism* 45:9 (1996): 1130–1135.

Brilla, L.R., and V. Conte. "Effects of Zinc-magnesium Formulation Increases Anabolic Hormones and Strength in Athletes." *Med Sci Sports Exerc* 31:5 (1999): 483.

Broca, C., R. Gross, P. Petit, et al. "4-Hydroxyisoleucine: Experimental Evidence of Its Insulinotropic and Antidiabetic Properties." *Am J Physiol* 277:4 Part 1 (1999): E617–E623.

ChemiNutraceutical in-house pilot study data (2003).

Czeisler, C., and E.B. Klerman. "Circadian and Sleep-dependent Regulation of Hormone Release in Humans." *Recent Prog Horm Res* 54 (1999): 97–130.

Di Luigi, L., L. Guidetti, F. Pigozzi, et al. "Acute Amino Acids Supplementation Enhances Pituitary Responsiveness in Athletes." *Med Sci Sports Exerc* 31:12 (1999): 1748–1754.

Dolezal, B.A., and J.A. Potteiger. "Concurrent Resistance and Endurance Training Influence Basal Metabolic Rate in Nondieting Individuals." *J Appl Physiol* 85:2 (1998): 695–700.

Fawcett, J.P., S.J. Farquhar, R.J. Walker, et al. "The Effect of Oral Vanadyl Sulfate on Body Composition and Performance in Weight-training Athletes." *Int J Sport Nutr* 6:4 (1996): 382–390.

Ghigo, E., E. Arvat, and F. Camanni. "Orally Active Growth Hormone Secretagogues: State of the Art and Clinical Perspectives." *Ann Med* 30:2 (1998): 159–168.

Gopal, K., R.K. Saran, S. Nityanand, et al. "Clinical Trial of Ethyl Acetate Extract of Gum Gugulu (Gugulipid) in Primary Hyperlipidemia." *J Assoc Physicians India* 34:4 (1986): 249–251.

Grant, K.E., R.M. Chandler, A.L. Castle, et al. "Chromium and Exercise Training: Effect on Obese Women." *Med Sci Sports Exerc* 29 (1997): 992–998.

Ikeda, Y. "The Clinical Study on the Water Extract of Leaves of *Lagerstroemia speciosa L* for Mild Cases of Diabetes Mellitus." Tokyo: Jikeikai University, 1998 (pilot study data).

Interhealth pilot study data (1998).

Jamieson, J., L. Dorman, and V. Marriot. *Growth Hormone: Reversing Human Aging Naturally.* East Canaan, CT: Safe Goods, 1997.

Johnston, C.S., C.S. Day, and P.D. Swan. "Postprandial Thermogenesis is Increased 100% on a High-protein, Low-fat Diet versus a High-carbohydrate, Low-fat Diet in Healthy, Young Women." *J Am Coll Nutr* 21:1 (2002): 55–61.

Kanaley, J.A., J.Y. Weltman, K.S. Pieper, et al. "Cortisol and Growth Hormone Responses to Exercise at Different Times of the Day." *J Clin Endocrinol Metab* 86:6 (2001): 2881–2889.

Kelley, D., et al. "Energy Restriction and Immunocompetence in Overweight Women." *Nutrition Research* 18:2 (1998): 159–169.

Lambert, M.I., J.A. Hefer, R.P. Millar, et al. "Failure of Commercial Oral Amino Acid Supplements to Increase Serum Growth Hormone Concentrations in Male Bodybuilders." *Int J Sport Nutr* 3:3 (1993): 298–305.

LeBlanc, J., I. Mercier, and A. Nadeau. "Components of Postprandial Thermogenesis in Relation to Meal Frequency in Humans." *Can J Physiol Pharmacol* 71:12 (1993): 879–883.

Madar, Z., et al. "Glucose-lowering Effect of Fenugreek in Non-insulin Dependent Diabetics." *Eur J Clin Nutr* 42:1 (1988): 51–54.

McCargar, L.J., and S.M. Crawford. "Metabolic and Anthropometric Changes with Weight Cycling in Wrestlers." *Med Sci Sports Exerc* 24:11 (1992): 1270-1275.

McMurray, R., T.K. Eubank, and A.C. Hackney. "Nocturnal Hormonal Responses to Resistance Exercise." *Eur J Appl Physiol Occup Physiol* 72:1-2 (1995): 121-126.

Mendelson, W. *Human Sleep.* New York: Plenum Press, 1989.

Monteleone, P., M. Maj, L. Beinat, et al. "Blunting by Chronic Phosphatidylserine Administration of the Stress-induced Activation of the Hypothalamo-pituitary-adrenal Axis in Healthy Men." *Eur J Clin Pharmacol* 42:4 (1992): 385–388.

Monteleone, P., L. Beinat, C. Tanzillo, et al. "Effects of Phosphatidylserine on the Neuroendocrine Responses to Physical Stress in Humans." *Neuroendocrinol* 52:3 (1990): 243–248.

Narayanan, C. "Pinitol—A New Anti-Diabetic Compound From the Leaves of Bougainvillea." *Current Science* 56:3 (1987): 139–141.

Nazar, K., A.W. Zemba, B. Kruk, et al. "Phosphate Supplementation Prevents a Decrease of Triiodothyronine and Increases Resting Metabolic Rate During Low Energy Diet." *J Physiol Pharmacol* 47:2 (1996): 373–383.

Ng, T.B., C.M. Wong, W.W. Li, et al. "Insulin-like Molecules in *Momordica charantia* Seeds." *J Ethnopharmacol* 15:1 (1986): 107–117.

Nindl, B.C., W.C. Hymer, D.R. Deaver, et al. "Growth Hormone Pulsatility Profile Characteristics Following Acute Heavy Resistance Exercise." *J Appl Physiol* 91:1 (2001): 163–172.

Nityanand, S., J.S. Srivastava, and O.P. Asthana. "Clinical Trials with Gugulipid. A New Hypolipidaemic Agent." *J Assoc Physicians India* 37:5 (1989): 323–328.

Pandey, S.K., M.B. Anand-Srivastava, and A.K. Srivastava. "Vanadyl Sulfate–stimulated Glycogen Synthesis is Associated with Activation of Phosphatidylinositol 3-kinase and is Independent of Insulin Receptor Tyrosine Phosphorylation." *Biochemistry* 37:19 (1998): 7006–7014.

Peters, E.M., R. Anderson, D.C. Nieman, et al. "Vitamin C Supplementation Attenuates the Increases in Circulating Cortisol, Adrenaline and Anti-inflammatory Polypeptides Following Ultramarathon Running." *Int J Sports Med* 22:7 (2001): 537–543.

Porchezhian, E., and R.M. Dobriyal. "An Overview on the Advances of *Gymnema sylvestre:* Chemistry, Pharmacology and Patents." *Pharmazie* 58:1 (2003): 5–12.

Rogers, N.L., M.P. Szuba, J.P. Staab, et al. "Neuroimmunologic Aspects of Sleep and Sleep Loss." *Semin Clin Neuropsychiatry* 6:4 (2001): 295–307.

Van Cauter, E., R. Leproult, and L. Plat. "Age-related Changes in Slow Wave Sleep and REM Sleep and Relationship with Growth Hormone and Cortisol Levels in Healthy Men." *JAMA* 284:7 (2000): 861–868.

Volek, J.S., W.J. Kraemer, J.A. Bush, et al. "Testosterone and Cortisol in Relationship to Dietary Nutrients and Resistance Exercise." *J Appl Physiol* 82:1 (1997): 49–54.

Welihinda, J., E.H. Karunanayake, M.H. Sheriff, et al. "Effect of *Momordica charantia* on the Glucose Tolerance in Maturity Onset Diabetes." *J Ethnopharmacol* 17:3 (1986): 277–282.

Weltman, A., J.Y. Weltman, J.D. Veldhuis, et al. "Body Composition, Physical Exercise, Growth Hormone and Obesity." *Eat Weight Disord* 6:3 Suppl (2001): 28–37.

Yan, W., K. Ohtani, R. Kasai, et al. "Steroidal Saponins from Fruits of *Tribulus terrestris.*" *Phytochemistry* 42:5 (1996): 1417–1422.

Chapter 5: Vitamins and Minerals for Optimal Health

Alaswad, K., J.H. O'Keefe Jr., and R.M. Moe. "Combination Drug Therapy for Dyslipidemia." *Curr Atheroscler Rep* 1:1 (1999): 44–49.

Aprahamian, M., A. Dentinger, C. Stock-Damge, et al. "Effects of Supplemental Pantothenic Acid on Wound Healing: Experimental Study in Rabbits." *Am J Clin Nutr* 41:3 (1985): 578–589.

Bender, D.A. *Nutritional Biochemistry of the Vitamins.* New York: Cambridge University Press, 1992, pp. 184–222.

Bhathena, S.J., L. Recant, N.R. Voyles, et al. "Decreased Plasma Enkephalins in Copper Deficiency in Man." *Am J Clin Nutr* 43:1 (1986): 42–46.

Brilla, L.R., and T.F. Haley. "Effect of Magnesium Supplementation on Strength Training in Humans." *J Amer Coll Nutr* 11:3 (1992): 326–329.

Cook, J.D., and E.R. Monson. "Vitamin C, The Common Cold, and Iron Absorption." *Am J Clin Nutr* 30 (1977): 235–241.

Cordova, A., and M. Alvarez-Mon. "Behavior of Zinc in Physical Exercise: A Special Reference to Immunity and Fatigue." *Neurosci Biobehav Rev* 19:3 (1995): 439–445.

Englisch, R., et al. "Induction of Glucose Transport into Rat Muscle by Selenate and Selenite: Comparison to Insulin." *Diabetologia* 38:1 Suppl (1995): A133.

Groff, J., S. Gropper, and S. Hunt. *Advanced Nutrition and Human Metabolism,* 2nd ed. St. Paul, MN: West, 1995.

Heyliger, C.E., A.G. Tahiliani, and J.H. McNeill. "Effect of Vanadate on Elevated Blood Glucose and Depressed Cardiac Performance of Diabetic Rats." *Science* 227 (1985): 1474–1477.

Johnston, C.S., and B. Luo. "Comparison of the Absorption and Excretion of Three Commercially Available Sources of Vitamin C." *J Am Diet Assoc* 94 (1994): 779–781.

Katts, G., et al. "The Effects of Chromium Picolinate Supplementation on Body Composition in Different Age Groups." *Age* 14:40 (1991): 138.

Kiremidjian-Schumacher, L., and G. Stotzky. "Selenium and Immune Responses." *Environmental Res* 42:2 (1987): 277–303.

Klesges, R.C., K.D. Ward, M.L. Shelton, et al. "Changes in Bone Mineral Content in Male Athletes: Mechanisms of Action and Intervention Effects." *JAMA* 276:3 (1996): 226–230.

Lemann, J., J.A. Pless, and R.W. Gary. "Potassium Causes Calcium Retention in Healthy Adults." *J Nutr* 123 (1993): 1623–1626.

Liakakos, D., N.L. Doulas, D. Ikkos, et al. "Inhibitory Effect of Ascorbic Acid (Vitamin C) on Cortisol Secretion Following Adrenal Stimulation in Children." *Clin Chem Acta* 65:3 (1975): 251–255.

Meador, K.J. "Evidence for a Central Cholinergic Effect of High-dose Thiamine." *Ann Neurol* 34 (1993): 724–726.

Peters, E.M., R. Anderson, D.C. Nieman, et al. "Vitamin C Supplementation Attenuates the Increases in Circulating Cortisol, Adrenaline and Anti-inflammatory Polypeptides Following Ultramarathon Running." *Int J Sports Med* 22:7 (2001): 537–543.

Phillips, C.L., S.B. Combs, and S.R. Pinnell. "Effects of Ascorbic Acid on Proliferation and Collagen Synthesis in Relation to the Donor Age of Human Dermal Fibroblasts." *J Invest Dermatol* 103:2 (1994): 228–232.

Prasad, A.S., C.S. Mantzoros, F.W. Beck, et al. "Zinc Status and Serum Testosterone Levels of Healthy Adults." *Nutrition* 12:5 (1996): 344–348.

Rupp, J.C., et al. "Effect of Sodium Bicarbonate Ingestion on Blood and Muscle pH and Exercise Performance." *Med Sci Sports Exerc* 15 (1983): 115.

Suttie, J.W. "Vitamin K and Human Nutrition." *J Am Diet Assoc* 92 (1992): 585-590.

Tufts University Health and Nutrition Letter 18:1 (2000).

Wilkes, D., N. Gledhill, and R. Smyth. "Effect of Induced Metabolic Alkalosis on 800-m Racing Time." *Med Sci Sports Exerc* 15:4 (1983): 277–280.

Wolf, G. "Multiple Functions of Vitamin A." *Physiol Rev* 64 (1984): 873–937.

Zemel, M.B. "Role of Dietary Calcium and Dairy Products in Modulating Adiposity." *Lipids* 38:2 (2003): 139–146.

Chapter 6: The Six-Pack Training Program

Bryner, R.W., R.C. Toffle, I.H. Ullrich, et al. "The Effects of Exercise Intensity on Body Composition, Weight Loss, and Dietary Composition in Women." *J Am Coll Nutr* 16:1 (1997): 68–73.

Dolezal, B.A., and J.A. Potteiger. "Concurrent Resistance and Endurance Training Influence Basal Metabolic Rate in Nondieting Individuals." *J Appl Physiol* 85:2 (1998): 695–700.

Durand, R.J., V.D. Castracane, D.B. Hollander, et al. "Hormonal Responses from Concentric and Eccentric Muscle Contractions." *Med Sci Sports Exerc* 35:6 (2003): 937–943.

Felsing, N.E., J.A. Brasel, and D.M. Cooper. "Effect of Low- and High-intensity Exercise on Circulating Growth Hormone in Men." *J Clin Endocrinol Metab* 75:1 (1992): 157–162.

Goto, K., K. Sato, and K. Takamatsu. "A Single Set of Low-intensity Resistance Exercise Immediately Following High-intensity Resistance Exercise Stimulates Growth Hormone Secretion in Men." *J Sports Med Phys Fitness* 43:2 (2003): 243–249.

Gotshalk, L.A., C.C. Loebel, B.C. Nindl, et al. "Hormonal Responses of Multiset versus Single-set Heavy-resistance Exercise Protocols." *Can J Appl Physiol* 22:3 (1997): 244–255.

Ivy, J.L. "Muscle Glycogen Synthesis Before and After Exercise." *Sports Med* 11:1 (1991): 6–19.

Kraemer, W.J., S.J. Fleck, J.E. Dziados, et al. "Changes in Hormonal Concentrations After Different Heavy-resistance Exercise Protocols in Women." *J Appl Physiol* 75:2 (1993): 594–604.

Naveri, H. "Blood Hormone and Metabolite Levels During Graded Cycle Ergometer Exercise." *Scand J Clin Lab Invest* 45:7 (1985): 599–603.

Putting It All Together

Addolorato, G., E. Capristo, A.V. Greco, et al. "Influence of Chronic Alcohol Abuse on Body Weight and Energy Metabolism: Is Excess Ethanol Consumption a Risk Factor for Obesity or Malnutrition?" *J Intern Med* 244:5 (1998): 387–395.

Dallongeville, J., N. Marecaux, P. Ducimetiere, et al. "Influence of Alcohol Consumption and Various Beverages on Waist Girth and Waist-to-hip Ratio in a Sample of French Men and Women." *Int J Obes Relat Metab Disord* 22:12 (1998): 1178–1183.

Mourier, A., A.X. Bigard, E. de Kerviler, et al. "Combined Effects of Caloric Restriction and Branched-chain Amino Acid Supplementation on Body Composition and Exercise Performance in Elite Wrestlers." *Int J Sports Med* 18:1 (1997): 47–55.

Pedersen, S.B., J.M. Bruun, F. Hube, et al. "Demonstration of Estrogen Receptor Subtypes Alpha and Beta in Human Adipose Tissue: Influences of Adipose Cell Differentiation and Fat Deposit Localization." *Mol Cell Endocrinol* 182:1 (2001): 27–37.

Riserus, U., L. Berglund, and B. Vessby. "Conjugated Linoleic Acid (CLA) Reduced Abdominal Adipose Tissue in Obese Middle-aged Men with Signs of the Metabolic Syndrome: A Randomised Controlled Trial." *Int J Obes Relat Metab Disord* 25:8 (2001): 1129–1135.

Index

About the Author

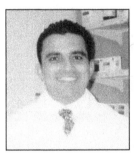

Rehan Jalali is founder and president of the Supplement Research Foundation (www.tsrf.com). He has been studying the science, efficacy, and safety of sports supplements for over ten years. He is a nationally recognized sports nutritionist who has developed over 100 cutting-edge products for the dietary supplement industry. Rehan has worked with and helped formulate products used by dozens of Olympic and professional athletes and celebrities, including Sylvester Stallone, Michael Strahan of the New York Giants, baseball players Turk Wendell and Benny Agbayani, boxer Shannon Briggs, Olympic Gold medalist Natalie Williams, world-class sprinter Dwight Thomas, and the Utah Jazz and New York Mets organizations. Rehan is also a natural bodybuilder who has held numerous bodybuilding titles, including Mr. Texas and the Ironman Natural Bodybuilding Champion.

Rehan is the author of *The Ultimate Performance Guide to Fitness Success* and co-author of *The Bodybuilding Supplement Guide.* He is a regular contributor to *Physical* magazine, *Health Products Business, Muscle Media,* and *Vitamin Retailer* and has published over 250 articles on nutrition and supplementation. His work as a writer, fitness expert, and fitness model has appeared in *Newsweek, Muscle and Fitness, Men's Health, Men's Fitness, Ironman Magazine, The Washington Post, MuscleMag International, Oxygen, Whole Foods Magazine, Real Solutions, Olympian's News, Personal Fitness Professional,* and *thinkmuscle.com,* among others. He is a nationally recognized speaker on nutrition, supplementation, and training.